Coagulation and Hematology in Neurological Surgery

Editors

SHAHID M. NIMJEE
RUSSELL R. LONSER

NEUROSURGERY CLINICS OF NORTH AMERICA

www.neurosurgery.theclinics.com

Consulting Editors
RUSSELL R. LONSER
DANIEL K. RESNICK

October 2018 • Volume 29 • Number 4

ELSEVIER

1600 John F. Kennedy Boulevard • Suite 1800 • Philadelphia, Pennsylvania, 19103-2899

http://www.theclinics.com

NEUROSURGERY CLINICS OF NORTH AMERICA Volume 29, Number 4
October 2018 ISSN 1042-3680, ISBN-13: 978-0-323-64091-6

Editor: Stacy Eastman
Developmental Editor: Laura Fisher

Neurosurgery Clinics of North America (ISSN 1042-3680) is published quarterly by Elsevier Inc., 360 Park Avenue South, New York, NY 10010-1710. Months of issue are January, April, July, and October. Business and Editorial Offices: 1600 John F. Kennedy Blvd., Suite 1800, Philadelphia, PA 19103-2899. Customer Service Office: 11830 Westline Industrial Drive, St. Louis, MO 63146. Periodicals postage paid at New York, NY, and additional mailing offices. Subscription prices are $417.00 per year (US individuals), $711.00 per year (US institutions), $449.00 per year (Canadian individuals), $884.00 per year (Canadian institutions), $505.00 per year (international individuals), $884.00 per year (international institutions), $100.00 per year (US students), and $255.00 per year (international and Canadian students). International air speed delivery is included in all *Clinics* subscription prices. All prices are subject to change without notice. **POSTMASTER:** Send address changes to *Neurosurgery Clinics of North America*, Elsevier Periodicals Customer Service, 11830 Westline Industrial Drive, St. Louis, MO 63146. **Customer Service: 1-800-654-2452 (US and Canada). From outside the US and Canada, call: 1-314-453-7041. Fax: 1-314-453-5170. E-mail: JournalsCustomerService-usa@elsevier.com (for print support) and journalsonlinesupport-usa@elsevier.com (for online support).**

Reprints. For copies of 100 or more, of articles in this publication, please contact the Commercial Reprints Department, Elsevier Inc., 360 Park Avenue South, New York, NY 10010-1710. Tel. 212-633-3874; Fax: 212-633-3820; E-mail: reprints@elsevier.com.

Neurosurgery Clinics of North America is covered in *MEDLINE/PubMed (Index Medicus)*, *EMBASE/Excerpta Medica*, and *Current Contents/Clinical Medicine (CC/CM)*.

Contributors

CONSULTING EDITORS

RUSSELL R. LONSER, MD
Professor and Chair, Department of
Neurological Surgery, The Ohio State
University Wexner Medical Center, Columbus,
Ohio, USA

DANIEL K. RESNICK, MD, MS
Professor and Vice Chairman, Program Director,
Department of Neurosurgery, University of
Wisconsin-Madison School of Medicine and
Public Health, Madison, Wisconsin, USA

EDITORS

SHAHID M. NIMJEE, MD, PhD
Associate Professor, Department of
Neurological Surgery, The Ohio State
University Wexner Medical Center, Columbus,
Ohio, USA

RUSSELL R. LONSER, MD
Professor and Chair, Department of
Neurological Surgery, The Ohio State University
Wexner Medical Center, Columbus, Ohio, USA

AUTHORS

GURSANT S. ATWAL, MD
Endovascular Neurosurgery Fellow,
Department of Neurosurgery, Jacobs School
of Medicine and Biomedical Sciences,
University at Buffalo, Department of
Neurosurgery, Gates Vascular Institute at
Kaleida Health, Buffalo, New York,
USA

MICHAL BAR-NATAN, MD
Division of Hematology and Oncology,
Department of Internal Medicine, Fellow, Laura
and Isaac Perlmutter Cancer Center, New York
University School of Medicine, New York,
New York, USA

JUSTIN BAUM, MD
Resident, Department of Neurological
Surgery, The Ohio State University
Wexner Medical Center, Columbus, Ohio,
USA

RICHARD C. BECKER, MD
Department of Medicine, Mabel Stonehill
Endowed Professor of Medicine, University of
Cincinnati Heart, Lung and Vascular Institute,
University of Cincinnati College of Medicine,
Cincinnati, Ohio, USA

TSINSUE CHEN, MD
Assistant Professor, Department of
Neurosurgery, Barrow Neurological Institute,
St Joseph's Hospital and Medical Center,
Phoenix, Arizona, USA

MADELEINE DE LOTBINIÈRE-BASSETT, MD
Division of Neurosurgery, Neurosurgery
Resident, Department of Clinical
Neurosciences, University of Calgary, Foothills
Hospital, Calgary, Alberta, Canada

TRACY A. DeWALD, PharmD, MHS
Clinical Pharmacist, Department of Medicine,
Duke Heart Center, Durham, North Carolina,
USA

DAVID DORNBOS III, MD
Chief Resident, Department of Neurological
Surgery, The Ohio State University Wexner
Medical Center, Columbus, Ohio, USA

AMMON M. FAGER, MD, PhD
Assistant Professor, Division of Hematology,
Department of Medicine, Duke University,
Division of Hematology/Oncology, Durham
Veterans Affairs Medical Center, Durham,
North Carolina, USA

GERALD A. GRANT, MD
Professor, Department of Neurosurgery,
Stanford University Medical Center, Stanford,
California, USA

MARK HAMILTON, MDCM, FRCSC, FAANS
Director, Adult Hydrocephalus Program,
Professor, Division of Neurosurgery,
Department of Clinical Neurosciences,
University of Calgary, Chair, Adult
Hydrocephalus Clinical Research Network,
Foothills Hospital, Calgary, Alberta,
Canada

MAUREANE HOFFMAN, MD, PhD
Professor, Department of Pathology,
Duke University, Pathology and Laboratory
Medicine Service, Durham Veterans Affairs
Medical Center, Durham, North Carolina,
USA

KENNETH B. HYMES, MD
Division of Hematology and Oncology,
Department of Internal Medicine, Associate
Professor, Laura and Isaac Perlmutter
Cancer Center, New York University School
of Medicine, New York, New York,
USA

ELAD I. LEVY, MD, MBA
L. Nelson Hopkins III, MD, Professor and
Chair of Neurosurgery, Departments of
Neurosurgery and Radiology, Jacobs School
of Medicine and Biomedical Sciences, Canon
Stroke and Vascular Research Center,
University at Buffalo, Department of
Neurosurgery, Gates Vascular Institute
at Kaleida Health, Buffalo, New York,
USA

CHRISTOPHER M. LOFTUS, MD
Professor, Department of Neurosurgery,
Lewis Katz School of Medicine,
Temple University, Temple University
Hospital, Philadelphia, Pennsylvania,
USA

RUSSELL R. LONSER, MD
Professor and Chair, Department of
Neurological Surgery, The Ohio State
University Wexner Medical Center, Columbus,
Ohio, USA

**ROBERT LOCH MACDONALD, MD, PhD,
FRCSC, FAANS, FACS**
Professor of Surgery, Division of Neurosurgery,
Departments of Surgery and Physiology,
St. Michael's Hospital, Labatt Family Centre
of Excellence in Brain Injury and Trauma
Research, Keenan Research Centre for
Biomedical Science, Li Ka Shing Knowledge
Institute, St. Michael's Hospital, University of
Toronto, Toronto, Ontario, Canada

HANH P. MAI, DO
Assistant Professor of Medicine, Department
of Hematology and Oncology, Loyola
University Medical Center, Maywood, Illinois,
USA

PETER NAKAJI, MD
Professor of Neurosurgery, Department of
Neurosurgery, Barrow Neurological Institute,
St Joseph's Hospital and Medical Center,
Phoenix, Arizona, USA

SUCHA NAND, MD
Professor of Medicine, Department of
Hematology and Oncology, Loyola University
Medical Center, Maywood, Illinois, USA

ARJUN NATARAJAN, MBBS, MD
Resident Physician, Department of Internal
Medicine, Advocate Illinois Masonic Medical
Center, Chicago, Illinois, USA

SHAHID M. NIMJEE, MD, PhD
Associate Professor, Department of
Neurological Surgery, The Ohio State
University Wexner Medical Center, Columbus,
Ohio, USA

JOEL Z. PASSER, MD
Resident, Department of Neurosurgery,
Temple University Hospital, Philadelphia,
Pennsylvania, USA

AUGUSTUS J. PEREZ, MD
Fellow, Pediatric Neurosurgery, Department of
Neurosurgery, Stanford University Medical
Center, Stanford, California, USA

GEORGE M. RODGERS, MD, PhD
Professor, Medicine, Pathology, Division of
Hematology and Hematologic Malignancies,
University of Utah Health Sciences Center, Salt
Lake City, Utah, USA

NICHOLAS SADER, MD
Neurosurgery Resident, Division of
Neurosurgery, Department of Clinical
Neurosciences, University of Calgary,
Foothills Hospital, Calgary, Alberta,
Canada

AMMAR SHAIKHOUNI, MD, PhD
Resident, Department of Neurological Surgery,
The Ohio State University Wexner Medical
Center, Columbus, Ohio, USA

DAULATH SINGH, MD
Fellow, Department of Hematology and
Oncology, Loyola University Medical Center,
Maywood, Illinois, USA

MICHAEL K. TSO, MD
Neurosurgery Resident, Division of
Neurosurgery, Department of Clinical
Neurosciences, University of Calgary,
Foothills Hospital, Calgary, Alberta,
Canada

KUNAL VAKHARIA, MD
Endovascular Neurosurgery Fellow,
Department of Neurosurgery, Jacobs School
of Medicine and Biomedical Sciences,
University at Buffalo, Department of
Neurosurgery, Gates Vascular Institute at
Kaleida Health, Buffalo, New York, USA

JEFFREY B. WASHAM, PharmD
Clinical Pharmacist, Department of Medicine,
Duke Heart Center, Durham, North Carolina,
USA

AMANDA S. ZAKERI, MD
Resident, Department of Neurological Surgery,
The Ohio State University Wexner Medical
Center, Columbus, Ohio, USA

JAMES J. ZHOU, MD
Resident, Department of Neurosurgery,
Barrow Neurological Institute, St. Joseph's
Hospital and Medical Center, Phoenix, Arizona,
USA

Contents

Section I: Biology and Evaluation

Hemostasis is a cell-based process that is regulated in a tissue-specific manner by the differential expression of procoagulant and anticoagulant factors on endothelial cells from different sites throughout the vasculature. The central nervous system, in particular, exhibits unique mechanisms of hemostatic regulation that favor increased activity of the tissue factor pathway. This results in an unusually high degree of protection against hemorrhage, at the potential expense of increased thrombotic risk. Unfortunately, standard laboratory assays, including the PT and aPTT, do not accurately reflect the complexity of hemostasis in vivo; therefore, they cannot predict the risk of bleeding or thrombosis.

Normal hemostasis provides for balanced interactions among the blood vessel wall, coagulation proteins, and platelets. After vascular injury, primary hemostasis and secondary hemostasis function in a coordinated fashion to stop bleeding. Standard coagulation tests have been shown in multiple studies to predict bleeding and mortality in neurosurgical patients. Emerging coagulation tests are useful point-of-care assays that guide transfusion therapy and diagnose patients with hyperfibrinolysis. This article provides an overview of hemostasis, a summary of standard coagulation testing and point-of-care tests, and a brief review of coagulation test usefulness in neurosurgery, focusing on studies in patients with traumatic brain injury.

Hemostasis is the normal process of blood coagulation in vivo to stop pathologic bleeding. Virchow triad includes venous stasis, hypercoagulability, and vascular injury. Natural anticoagulants include protein C, protein S, and antithrombin. Factor V Leiden is the most common inherited thrombophilia, followed by prothrombin gene mutation. All inherited thrombophilias are passed down in an autosomal dominant fashion. Patients harboring the antiphospholipid antibodies have an increased risk for thrombosis. von Willebrand disease is the most common inherited bleeding disorder; the pattern of inheritance is autosomal. Hemophilia A and B are the only hereditary bleeding disorders inherited in a sex-linked recessive pattern.

Section II: Anticoagulants

Anticoagulant medications are used widely for a variety of medical and surgical diseases, disorders, and conditions associated with thrombosis and thromboembolism. This article highlights labeled indications, mechanisms of action, potential drug interactions, and specific pharmacokinetic characteristics of available anticoagulants as an essential foundation for guiding selection and management of therapies for patients undergoing neurosurgical procedures.

Antiplatelet agents used to treat neurovascular disease include aspirin; P2Y12 receptor antagonists clopidogrel, prasugrel, and ticagrelor; ADP antagonist ticlopidine; phosphodiesterase inhibitor dipyridamole; and glycoprotein IIb/IIIa inhibitors abciximab, eptifibatide, and tirofiban. Numerous studies have been performed evaluating their efficacy in stroke, extracranial carotid artery disease and dissection, intracranial atherosclerotic disease, and moyamoya disease. The rapid technological advancements in endovascular neurosurgical devices have also made antiplatelet therapy a necessary part of treating intracranial aneurysms. This article presents the relevant data supporting the use of antiplatelet agents in vascular neurosurgery and recommendations based on the described studies.

Long-term anticoagulant therapy prevents thrombosis. Management of neurosurgical patients with conditions such as atrial fibrillation, mechanical heart valves, and other prothrombotic states necessitates application of a strategy to mitigate hemorrhagic complications of anticoagulation. Development of direct oral anticoagulants, which include the direct thrombin and factor X inhibitors, yields new considerations to be had, in particular, the introduction of reversal agents. This article reviews the more common chronic clinical entities that require the use of prolonged anticoagulant therapy with special consideration for neurosurgical patients. It also includes a discussion of established treatment strategies across available treatment options.

Although antiplatelet medications and anticoagulants are necessary for numerous cardiac comorbidities, prevention of stroke, and treatment and prevention of venous thromboembolic events, they pose a significant treatment dilemma in neurosurgical patients, particularly in the setting of intracranial hemorrhage or before emergent neurosurgical procedures. For most current anticoagulation and antiplatelet therapies, no direct reversal agents exist; however, there are numerous strategies that can be used to reverse or mitigate their antithrombotic properties. This article provides a comprehensive summary of the latest antiplatelet and anticoagulant therapies and the role of emergency reversal before emergent neurosurgical procedures.

Section III: Coagulation in the Perioperative Patient

Intraoperative blood and coagulation factor transfusion is of particular importance to neurosurgeons. Maintaining the hematologic and coagulation parameters of the patient within normal limits during surgery is critical to facilitate normal hemostasis, reduce transfusion requirements, and prevent complications associated with excessive blood loss. In this article, the authors review topics relevant to intraoperative transfusion during neurosurgery, including laboratory studies and other diagnostic modalities available to help with decision making, blood components and coagulation factors currently available for transfusion, and indications for intraoperative transfusion during cranial and spinal neurosurgical procedures.

Intraoperative bleeding can be minimized with optimal preoperative preparation but cannot be completely prevented. There are circumstances when patients need emergent operative intervention, and thorough hemostatic evaluation and preparation are not possible. In this article, the authors summarize the recommendations for rapid reversal of vitamin K antagonists and direct oral anticoagulants before procedures. The authors review the potential causes for intraoperative bleeding and the methods for rapid and accurate diagnosis. The authors summarize the current evidence for treatment options, including transfusion of platelets and coagulation factors and the use of topical agents, antidotes to direct-acting anticoagulants, antifibrinolytics, and desmopressin.

The optimal approach for deep vein thrombosis (DVT) prophylaxis in the neurosurgery patient is a challenge of balancing the reduction in incidence of DVT and pulmonary embolus (PE) without risking an increase in catastrophic hemorrhages. In this article, the authors review the current literature on DVT/PE prophylaxis in neurosurgery. Mechanical and pharmacologic DVT prophylaxis strategies are discussed in terms of their efficacy in reducing DVT/PE rates as well as safety in terms of catastrophic hemorrhages. The authors offer recommendations regarding the best approach given the current state of the literature.

Management of anticoagulation and antiplatelet medications after neurosurgery can be complex, especially given that these patients have multiple medical comorbidities. In turn, neurosurgical patients are at high risk for the development of venous thromboembolism after surgery, so neurosurgeons must consider the use of pharmacologic prophylaxis. Developments in endovascular neurosurgery have produced therapies that require close management of antiplatelet medications to prevent postoperative complications. Any of these patient populations may need intrathecal access. This article highlights current strategies for managing these issues in the neurosurgical patient population.

Section IV: Treatment of Thrombosis in the Neurosurgical Patient

Cerebral venous sinus thrombosis (CVST) is a rare subtype of cerebrovascular disease representing 0.5% of strokes. The signs and symptoms of CVST are often nonspecific, and variable in duration, with the common results being delayed diagnosis and treatment. Increased awareness in the medical community and advancements in imaging modalities have produced faster diagnosis with improved patient outcomes. The preferred initial treatment is with a low molecular weight heparin. After the acute stage of CVST, treatment with a vitamin K antagonist (oral anticoagulant therapy) is recommended. Current evidence suggests that in the future, factor Xa inhibitor drugs may be used for long-term therapy.

Acute ischemic thrombosis in patients who have undergone neurosurgical procedures is a leading cause of mortality and long-term disability. Endovascular therapy has become an important treatment modality for acute ischemic thrombosis in these patients. Noninvasive imaging has dramatically changed the understanding of cerebral blood flow and the concepts of cerebrovascular reserve and salvageable penumbra. Increasingly, reliance on perfusion imaging to discern tissue viability and potential outcomes has become standard of care. With the advent of recent acute ischemic stroke trials, therapy for occlusive cerebrovascular disease is evolving, and understanding when to intervene is becoming paramount.

Antiplatelet and anticoagulant drugs (antithrombotic drugs) can cause or be associated with intracranial hemorrhage. Patients who take antithrombotic drugs are at higher risk for intracranial hemorrhage after trauma and are neurologically worse acutely compared with patients not on antithrombotic drugs. Treatment of patients on antithrombotic drugs who have intracranial hemorrhage includes reversal of anticoagulant drugs in almost all cases. This article is a synopsis of the data pertaining to intracranial hemorrhage and antithrombotic drugs and methods to diagnose the pharmacologic effects and to reverse the effects of these drugs in patients with traumatic or spontaneous intracranial hemorrhage.

NEUROSURGERY CLINICS OF NORTH AMERICA

SERIES OF RELATED INTEREST

Neurologic Clinics
http://www.neurologicclinics.com
Neuroimaging Clinics
http://www.neuroimaging.theclinics.com/

THE CLINICS ARE AVAILABLE ONLINE!
Access your subscription at:
www.theclinics.com

Preface
Coagulation and Hematology in Neurologic Surgery

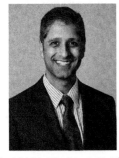 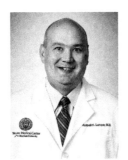

Shahid M. Nimjee, MD, PhD   Russell R. Lonser, MD
Editors

We sincerely appreciate the opportunity to serve as guest editors for this issue of *Neurosurgery Clinics of North America*, which focuses on coagulation and hematology as it pertains to the neurosurgical patient.

For decades, cardiovascular disease has been the leading cause of mortality in the United States, responsible for 1 out of every 3 deaths, while stroke is the leading cause of combined morbidity and mortality. Medical therapy includes antiplatelets, anticoagulants, and fibrinolytics. While they have improved outcomes affecting both groups of patients, their use poses challenges to the neurosurgeon, including understanding their indications, risk of hemorrhage, in terms of both spontaneous intracranial hemorrhage and surgical blood loss while patients are on these agents. With the relatively recent development of anti-FXa inhibitors and oral anti-thrombin inhibitors, this has become an even greater consideration. These new compounds, known as novel oral anticoagulants, don't require monitoring and demonstrate only a nominal increase in the usual coagulation parameters obtained prior to surgery. This potentially places the patient at increased risk of hemorrhage in the setting of a neurosurgical emergency. Fortunately, drug reversal strategies, including prothrombin complex concentrate, as well as drug-specific antidotes like Idarucizumab (Dabigatran antidote) and Andexinet alpha (FXa inhibitor antidote), are beginning to address some of theses challenges.

In this issue of *Neurosurgery Clinics of North America*, we have organized the information into four sections. The first section focuses on the molecular biology of coagulation and the role of coagulation factors and platelets in thrombus formation. We then describe how to evaluate coagulopathies in the neurosurgical patient and review genetic coagulopathies. The second section reviews the mechanism of anticoagulant and antiplatelet drugs, their use to treat disease, and reversal strategies in the setting of a neurosurgical emergency. Section three provides an overview of managing intraoperative blood loss and provides guidance on deep vein thrombosis prophylaxis and restarting systemic anticoagulation after a neurosurgical procedure. Finally, section four summarizes management of acute arterial and venous thrombosis in the brain and strategies to manage intracranial hemorrhage in the anticoagulated patient.

We hope that this issue provides neurosurgeons with a reference to understand how to appropriately use anticoagulant and antithrombotic drugs, their role in treating neurologic

Neurosurg Clin N Am 29 (2018) xiii–xiv
https://doi.org/10.1016/j.nec.2018.07.001
1042-3680/18/© 2018 Published by Elsevier Inc.

disease, and how to reverse them urgently or emergently for surgery.

Shahid M. Nimjee, MD, PhD
Department of Neurological Surgery
The Ohio State University
Wexner Medical Center
N-1014 Doan Hall
410 West 10th Avenue
Columbus, OH 43210, USA

Russell R. Lonser, MD
Department of Neurological Surgery
The Ohio State University
Wexner Medical Center
N-1047 Doan Hall
410 West 10th Avenue
Columbus, OH 43210, USA

E-mail addresses:
shahid.nimjee@osumc.edu (S.M. Nimjee)
russell.lonser@osumc.edu (R.R. Lonser)

Section I: Biology and Evaluation

Biology of Coagulation and Coagulopathy in Neurologic Surgery

Ammon M. Fager, MD, PhD[a,b],
Maureane Hoffman, MD, PhD[c,d],*

KEYWORDS

- Coagulation • Hemostasis • Thrombin • Fibrinolysis • Brain • Neurosurgery • Prothrombin time
- Partial thromboplastin time

KEY POINTS

- Hemostasis is cell-based and tightly regulated in a tissue-specific manner by differential expression of procoagulant and anticoagulant factors on endothelial cells from different sites throughout the vasculature.
- The brain exhibits unique mechanisms of hemostatic regulation that favor increased tissue factor pathway activity to protect against hemorrhage at the expense of increased thrombotic risk.
- Although the "cascade" model of coagulation is useful for interpreting the PT and aPTT assays, neither of these tests accurately reflects the complexity of hemostasis in vivo.

INTRODUCTION

Hemostasis is a tightly regulated process designed to prevent hemorrhage while maintaining the fluidity of blood in circulation. This process is dependent on interactions among platelets, endothelial cells, and plasma proteins that facilitate coagulation at sites of injury. Meanwhile, hemostasis is limited by the antithrombotic and fibrinolytic systems to prevent thrombosis and facilitate wound healing.

Although blood circulation allows effective communication and trafficking between organ systems, systemic alterations in hemostatic components invariably lead to localized rather than diffuse patterns of hemorrhage or thrombosis. This suggests that the process of hemostasis is regulated in a tissue-specific manner determined by the differential expression of procoagulant and anticoagulant properties within various tissue types.[1–3]

The purpose of this article is to (1) provide a general framework for understanding the process of hemostasis; (2) highlight unique regulatory mechanisms in the brain; and (3) review the limitations of laboratory testing in assessing hemostasis.

MECHANISMS OF HEMOSTASIS

The hemostatic response is divided into 2 concomitant and interdependent stages termed

Conflicts of Interest: The authors declare no conflicts of interest.
Sources of Funding: A.M. Fager is supported by a competitive investigator-initiated research grant from the Bayer Hemophilia Awards Program (Early Career Investigator Award). M. Hoffman is supported by the US Department of Veterans Affairs.
a Division of Hematology, Department of Medicine, Duke University, DUMC Box #3422, Durham, NC 27710, USA; b Division of Hematology/Oncology, Durham Veterans Affairs Medical Center, 508 Fulton Street, Durham, NC 27705, USA; c Department of Pathology, Duke University, DUMC Box #3712, Durham, NC 27710, USA; d Pathology and Laboratory Medicine Service, Durham Veterans Affairs Medical Center, 508 Fulton Street, Durham, NC 27705, USA
* Corresponding author. Pathology and Laboratory Medicine Service, Durham Veterans Affairs Medical Center, 508 Fulton Street, Durham, NC, 27705.
E-mail address: Maureane.hoffman@duke.edu

Neurosurg Clin N Am 29 (2018) 475–483
https://doi.org/10.1016/j.nec.2018.05.001
1042-3680/18/Published by Elsevier Inc.

primary and secondary hemostasis. Primary hemostasis is initiated by vascular injury leading to vasoconstriction and exposure of the subendothelial matrix. Platelets rapidly adhere to the site of injury where they undergo activation and aggregation to form a temporary platelet plug. Secondary hemostasis involves activation of the coagulation cascade to facilitate the production of thrombin in sufficient amounts to cleave fibrinogen and stabilize the platelet plug. In addition, thrombin triggers the anticoagulant and fibrinolytic systems that limit the hemostatic response while maintaining clot integrity long enough to ensure wound repair.

Early Models of Hemostasis

In 1905, Paul Morawitz[4] proposed the first biochemical model of coagulation in which thrombokinase, also known as thromboplastin or tissue factor (TF), converts prothrombin to thrombin in a calcium-dependent manner. In 1935, A.J. Quick[5] used this model to develop the initial prothrombin time (PT) to assay plasma levels of prothrombin. In 1953, the partial thromboplastin time (PTT) was developed to aid in the diagnosis of hemophilia.[6] It was later modified using kaolin as an activator to make it more rapid and reproducible. Thus, the activated PTT (aPTT) was born.[7]

As additional coagulation factors were discovered over the first half of the twentieth century, updated models of coagulation were needed to explain this increasingly complex system.

Results from the PT and aPTT assays contributed to the development of the waterfall or "cascade" model of coagulation in 1964.[8,9] In this model, each coagulation factor exists as a zymogen that is converted into an active enzyme by proteolytic cleavage. Coagulation occurs via a series of steps in which each factor activates the next. In this manner, a series of proteases acts as a biological amplifier that ultimately generates enough thrombin to produce a stable fibrin clot.

Subsequent modifications of the cascade model resulted in the now familiar Y-shaped scheme consisting of 2 distinct pathways that converge at the level of the prothrombinase (factor Xa [FXa]/FVa) complex (**Fig. 1**). In this scheme, the "intrinsic" pathway, so called because all components are present in plasma, is initiated by FXII. In contrast, the "extrinsic" pathway is initiated by FVIIa/TF and therefore requires a component that is normally external to the blood.

The cascade model was originally proposed to illustrate biochemical interactions between coagulation factors, and not as a literal model of hemostasis in vivo. Therefore, this model

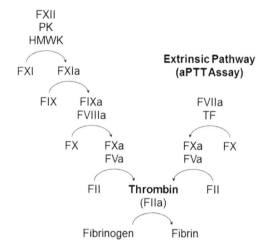

Intrinsic Pathway (PT Assay)

Extrinsic Pathway (aPTT Assay)

Fig. 1. The cascade model of coagulation. The intrinsic and extrinsic pathways converge at the FXa/FVa complex, which generates enough thrombin to cleave fibrinogen and form a mature clot. This model is an excellent tool for interpreting the aPTT and PT assays, which monitor factor levels in the intrinsic or extrinsic pathway, respectively. HMWK, high molecular weight kininogen; PK, prekallikrein.

does not include the anticoagulant pathways that provide both spatial and temporal regulation of thrombin formation. In addition, it cannot explain why a functional extrinsic pathway is unable to prevent bleeding in patients with hemophilia or other isolated defects of the intrinsic pathway. Despite these limitations, the cascade model provides an excellent tool for interpreting the PT and aPTT assays on which it was based.

A Cell-Based Model of Hemostasis

Since the discoveries of platelets[10] and the Virchow triad[11] in the mid-nineteenth century, cells have been widely recognized as important participants in coagulation. Thus, a current model of hemostasis incorporates the important role of cells that is lacking in the cascade model.[12]

According to the cell-based model, hemostasis occurs in a stepwise process on specific cell surfaces that differentially express procoagulant and anticoagulant proteins and receptors (**Fig. 2**). This process is divided into 3 overlapping stages: (1) initiation on the surface of a TF-bearing cell, (2) amplification, which sets the stage for large-scale thrombin generation, and (3) propagation on the platelet surface, which facilitates large-scale thrombin generation.

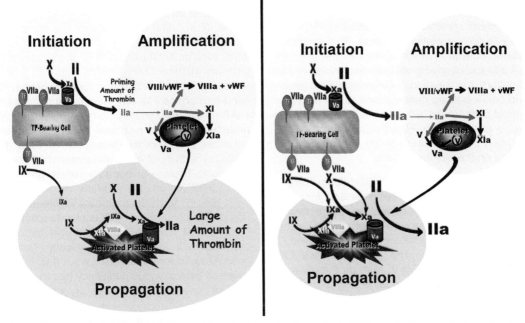

Fig. 2. A cell-based model of coagulation and its adaptation to the brain. Left: Hemostasis occurs in 3 overlapping stages. Initiation occurs on the surface of TF-bearing cells where FVIIa/TF activates FIX and FX. FXa binds FVa to generate small amounts of thrombin, which activates platelets and other coagulation factors in the amplification stage. During the propagation stage, thrombin is produced on the activated platelet surface in sufficiently large amounts to effect hemostasis. Right: Tissue-specific regulation in the brain is focused on protecting against hemorrhage and suggests that FVIIa/TF may play a greater role in thrombin generation during the propagation stage than it does in other tissues.

Stage 1: initiation on tissue factor-bearing cells

The hemostatic process begins with vascular injury and localized exposure of subendothelial collagen and extracellular matrix. Circulating platelets quickly adhere to the damaged area. This binding initiates intracellular signaling that results in partial platelet activation. The platelets then aggregate to form the primary platelet plug. Long-term hemostasis requires stabilization of this temporary platelet plug by a meshwork of fibrin that is formed by the thrombin-mediated cleavage of fibrinogen. In addition, thrombin activates FXIII, which cross-links the fibrin strands to form the mature clot.

The extrinsic pathway (FVIIa/TF) is the sole initiator of thrombin generation in vivo. Endothelial disruption exposes TF, which is highly expressed by pericytes and adventitial cells surrounding blood vessels.[13] Thus, TF contributes to a "hemostatic envelope" ready to activate coagulation in the event of tissue injury.[14]

Circulating FVII binds TF and is autoactivated to FVIIa.[15] The resulting FVIIa/TF complex can activate FIX to FIXa and FX to FXa.[16]

Meanwhile, activated platelets release a form of platelet-derived FVa at the site of injury.[17,18] This

FVa binds the newly generated FXa to form prothrombinase complexes that generate a small amount of thrombin on the surface of TF-bearing cells.[19] Although this thrombin is not sufficient to produce a stable fibrin clot, it is essential for fully activating platelets and other coagulation factors in the amplification stage.

In contrast to FXa, the FIXa activated by FVIIa/TF does not act on the surface of the TF-bearing cell. Instead, FIXa can diffuse to the surface of nearby activated platelets where it plays a significant role in the propagation stage.

Most coagulation factors can extravasate from the vasculature and collect in the lymph.[20] At sites around vessels, a significant proportion of TF is bound to FVII/FVIIa even in the absence of injury.[21] Therefore, it is likely that low levels of FIXa, FXa, and thrombin are produced constitutively on TF-bearing cells. However, this process is normally separated from other components of hemostasis by an intact vessel wall.

Stage 2: amplification

During the amplification stage, thrombin formed on TF-bearing cells accumulates to reach levels capable of promoting maximal platelet activation.[22] This thrombin also plays a critical role in "priming" the system for a subsequent burst of thrombin generation by activating FV, FVIII, and FXI on the platelet surface. The thrombin-induced activation of FXI abrogates the need for FXII and explains why severe deficiencies in FXII do not result in bleeding.[23] Meanwhile, FIXa generated on TF-bearing cells diffuses to the activated platelet surface where it binds to FVIIIa and forms the "tenase" complex (FIXa/FVIIIa). This process is amplified by the FXIa-mediated activation of FIX directly on the platelet surface.

Stage 3: propagation on the platelet surface

The large amount of thrombin necessary for effective hemostasis is produced on the activated platelet surface during the propagation stage. Once the FIXa/FVIIIa complex is assembled, it converts FX to FXa. The platelet-surface FXa then associates with FVa to form prothrombinase complexes capable of producing thrombin in sufficient amounts to cleave fibrinogen and yield a mature clot.[24]

The critical contribution of the platelet surface is highlighted by the severe bleeding diathesis seen in patients with deficiencies in FVIII (hemophilia A) or FIX (hemophilia B). Although FXIa is capable of enhancing FIXa production on platelets, this is not essential because FIXa produced on TF-bearing cells can diffuse to the platelet surface. Thus, FXI deficiency generally results in milder and more varied bleeding than hemophilia A or B.

Even though the cell-based model depicts hemostasis as occurring in discrete steps, these should be viewed as an overlapping continuum of events. For example, early in the propagation stage, thrombin produced on the platelet surface may activate additional coagulation factors for amplification of the response rather than leaving the platelet to promote fibrin assembly.

Based on this model, it is clear that the classical intrinsic and extrinsic pathways are not redundant. The extrinsic pathway operates on TF-bearing cells to initiate and amplify coagulation, whereas the intrinsic pathway acts on activated platelets to propagate large-scale thrombin production. Therefore, the PT tests the levels of factors involved in the initiation stage, whereas the aPTT tests the levels of factors involved in the propagation stage. As such, neither assay gives a complete picture of hemostatic function.

Coagulation Is Localized to Appropriate Surfaces

As illustrated previously, the process of hemostasis is tightly regulated both spatially and temporally to prevent hemorrhage while avoiding widespread thrombosis.

The appropriate localization of the hemostatic response is primarily ensured by circulating inhibitors, such as antithrombin (AT), and tissue factor pathway inhibitor (TFPI), which limit FXa activity to the surface on which it is formed; hence, the need to produce FXa on different cell surfaces.

AT (previously antithrombin III) is serpin-type protease inhibitor responsible for inactivating thrombin, FXa, and, to a lesser extent, FIXa. The inhibitory activity of AT is enhanced 1000-fold by binding to heparin or heparan sulfate proteoglycans (HSPG) on the surface of endothelial cells. Binding to HSPG promotes allosteric activation of AT. Long-chain HSPGs also function as a scaffold that binds AT and its target factors to promote their interaction.[25] Clinically, homozygous AT deficiency is almost always fatal in utero, whereas heterozygous deficiency has the highest risk of venous thrombosis of any inherited thrombophilia.[26]

TFPI is a Kunitz-type protease inhibitor expressed in 2 alternatively spliced isoforms, TFPIα and TFPIβ. Whereas TFPIα circulates in the blood and is secreted by activated platelets at sites of injury, TFPIβ remains tethered to the surface of endothelial cells.[27] TFPI is the primary inhibitor of the initiation stage because both isoforms inhibit FVIIa/TF and FXa. The inhibition of FXa by TFPI is enhanced ninefold in the presence of Protein S (PS); however, PS has no clear role in TFPI-mediated inhibition of FVIIa/TF.

TFPIα also acts as a potent inhibitor of prothrombinase complexes that contain FXa-activated or platelet-derived FVa. This ability is unique to TFPIα, is not enhanced by PS, and does not occur when prothrombinase contains thrombin-activated FVa. Therefore, although TFPIα can inhibit prothrombinase activity during the initiation stage, it has no effect during the propagation stage.[27]

Homozygous TFPI deficiency has not been described in humans, suggesting embryonic lethality. Conversely, heterozygous TFPI deficiency leads to an increased risk of venous[28] and arterial[29] thrombosis, including ischemic stroke.

The localization of AT and TFPI allows them to specifically inhibit coagulation factors in the plasma or on the endothelium. Although surface-bound FXa is relatively protected, FXa in solution is often inhibited within seconds.[30] Therefore, FXa activity remains limited to the cell surface on which it was formed. In contrast, FIXa can diffuse to nearby platelet surfaces because it is not inhibited by TFPI, and its AT-mediated inhibition is much less efficient than that of FXa.

The Protein C/S Pathway Protects Against Thrombosis

Inhibition of the FIXa/FVIIIa and FXa/FVa complexes during the propagation stage relies on the thrombin-initiated Protein C (PC) system.

As thrombin levels rise during propagation, some thrombin escapes from the site of injury and binds to thrombomodulin (TM), a cell surface receptor expressed on endothelial cells. Once bound to TM, thrombin is no longer procoagulant. Instead, thrombin/TM cleaves PC bound to endothelial cell protein C receptor (EPCR) and converts it to activated protein C (APC). APC then binds PS, and the APC/PS complex proteolytically inactivates FVa and FVIIIa on endothelial surfaces.

Although APC is often called an "anticoagulant," it does not normally act in the fluid phase and has limited ability to inactivate FVa on platelets.[31] Therefore, APC/PS does not normally "turn off" coagulation. Instead, it prevents thrombin generation and thrombosis on uninjured endothelium away from the site of injury.

Clinically, deficiencies in PC or PS lead to an increased risk of both arterial and venous thrombosis.[32] Conversely, excess activation of PC following trauma can contribute to a systemic coagulopathy.[33] In addition, APC binding to EPCR mediates anti-inflammatory and cytoprotective effects in a variety of diseases, including stroke, coronary reperfusion injury, and diabetes.[34]

The Fibrinolytic System Protects Against Thrombosis

The fibrinolytic system protects against thrombosis by degrading clots within intact vessels and by eliminating senescent clots during wound healing.

Plasmin is the key enzyme responsible for cleaving both fibrinogen and fibrin into soluble degradation products. Plasmin is produced from circulating plasminogen by 1 of 2 activators: urinary plasminogen activator (uPA, urokinase) or tissue plasminogen activator (tPA).

tPA is synthesized by endothelial cells and released in response to thrombin or hypoxia. uPA is produced by a variety of cell types. Although uPA effectively activates circulating plasminogen, tPA is far more effective when bound, with plasminogen, to the fibrin meshwork of a mature clot. uPA has therefore been suggested to play a larger role in preventing the intravascular deposition of fibrin associated with developing atherosclerosis, whereas tPA is routinely used as a therapeutic agent for lysing existing clots.

Both uPA and tPA are controlled by plasminogen activator inhibitor-1 (PAI-1), which is synthesized by a variety of cells, including endothelial cells and astrocytes. PAI-1 is also released from activated platelets to prevent premature clot dissolution.[35]

Clinically, PAI-1 has been suggested to play diverse roles in the evolution of brain damage and recovery after stroke.[36] In addition, elevated PAI-1 levels are associated with an increased risk of atherosclerosis and vascular thrombosis, whereas complete PAI-1 deficiency results in life-threatening hemorrhage and delayed wound healing.[36] Thus, effective hemostasis depends on appropriate fibrinolysis.

TISSUE-SPECIFIC REGULATION OF HEMOSTASIS

Based on the previously described models, systemic alterations in hemostatic components would be expected to cause diffuse thrombotic or hemorrhagic events throughout the body. Instead, such alterations almost invariably result in localized lesions, suggesting that hemostasis is regulated in a tissue-specific manner.[1–3]

This concept is supported by multiple murine studies.[3] For example, mice that lack tPA, uPA, or thrombomodulin exhibit increased fibrin deposition in various organs, but not in the brain.[37] Conversely, mice with low levels of TF or FVII showed spontaneous hemorrhages in the brain, while other organs were spared.[38] Studies using double knockout mice reveal entirely new patterns of localized dysfunction.[1]

Taken together, these data suggest that endothelial cell heterogeneity results in different site-specific strategies to mediate the local hemostatic balance within tissues. This is consistent with clinical observations that site-specific thrombosis occurs with various thrombophilias,[1] whereas tissue-specific patterns of hemorrhage occur with anticoagulants that target different coagulation factors.[39]

Regulation of Hemostasis in the Brain

Hemostasis is uniquely regulated in the central nervous system. Compared with other organs, the brain microvasculature is specifically designed to provide an unusually high degree of protection against hemorrhage, at the potential expense of increased thrombotic risk.[2]

Structural regulation

The blood-brain barrier is dependent on characteristic tight junctions between endothelial cells in the cerebral capillaries. These tight junctions provide protection against hemorrhage that goes well beyond the normal adherens junctions in the systemic microvasculature.[40]

In addition, pericytes are preferentially localized directly opposite capillary tight junctions to form an additional barrier that enhances the protection against hemorrhage. Pericytes are also capable of erythrophagocytosis to prevent erythrocyte egress, and their localization facilitates the paracrine production of trophic factors that further enhance the blood-brain barrier.[41]

Functional regulation of coagulation

The functional components of hemostasis and its regulatory pathways are expressed in a tissue-specific manner by endothelial cells, pericytes, and astrocytes in the cerebral microvasculature.

The brain is a particularly rich source of TF,[14] which is highly expressed by astrocytes[42] and pericytes[43] throughout the cortex. Indeed, approximately 800 million PT assays are performed annually using TF derived largely from brain extracts.[44] Furthermore, unlike dermal vessels, the brain contains high amounts of "free" TF, which is not bound to FVII/FVIIa.[45] Therefore, the optimal dose of FVIIa for management of intracerebral hemorrhage may be considerably lower than for bleeding at non–central nervous system sites.[45]

In contrast, although TFPI is measurably expressed by cerebral endothelial cells, astrocytes, and oligodendrocytes, this expression is lower in the brain than all other organs tested.[46] Furthermore, the inhibitory activity of AT is dependent on binding to HSPGs on the endothelial cell surface. Despite being widely expressed in most tissues, HSPGs are not expressed in cerebral capillaries.[47] Thus, the anticoagulant effect of AT is also significantly downregulated in the brain.

High levels of TF combined with low levels of TFPI and AT suggest that the activity of the FVIIa/TF pathway is increased in the brain, where it likely plays a greater role in thrombin generation during the propagation stage than it does in other tissues (see **Fig. 2**). This is supported by the observation that nontraumatic intracerebral bleeding is relatively rare with severe acute thrombocytopenia.[48]

The activity of the PC/PS pathway is also downregulated by the very low expression of both TM[49,50] and EPCR[51] in the brain. Because APC has both antithrombotic and cytoprotective effects that decrease tissue damage in spinal cord injury and stroke,[52] the decreased production of APC has important implications in both hemorrhage and thrombosis. This is supported by the observation that TM expression is particularly low in regions with a propensity to develop lacunar infarcts.[49]

Functional regulation of fibrinolysis

The fibrinolytic system is also differentially regulated by cerebral endothelial cells. For example, tPA expression is largely absent in the brain due to astrocyte-specific inhibition induced by blood-brain barrier formation.[50] Furthermore, although systemic endothelial cells release tPA in response to thrombin, cerebral endothelial cells do not. Instead, thrombin stimulation of cerebral endothelial cells leads to dose-dependent uPA secretion, suggesting that uPA is the major activator of fibrinolysis in the brain.[53] Because uPA activates plasminogen on binding sites exposed by tPA,[54] the net effect may be an overall delay in cerebral fibrinolysis, which contributes to a pro-hemostatic environment in the brain.

In addition, PAI-1 expression is enhanced in cerebral endothelial cells and astrocytes during formation of the blood-brain barrier.[50] This expression is further increased by thrombin stimulation. Thus, thrombin mediates an early increase in PAI-1 expression followed by a delayed increase in uPA that is likely designed to prevent premature dissolution of the clot.[53]

IMPLICATIONS FOR CLINICAL LABORATORY TESTING

Neither the cascade model nor the PT/aPTT assays it describes can accurately reflect the complexity of hemostasis in vivo. Therefore it is critical to understand the capabilities and limitations of these tests.

These assays were designed to confirm a suspected deficiency in one or more coagulation factors; however, these tests are significantly limited by technical factors, insensitivity to some bleeding disorders, and sensitivity to common abnormalities that carry no bleeding risk. Therefore, the PT and/or aPTT should not be used to predict clinical bleeding.[55]

For example, in laboratory practice, the "normal" range is usually defined as 2 standard deviations surrounding the mean of the normal population. Therefore, by definition, 2.5% of healthy subjects have a prolonged PT/aPTT.

In addition, life-threatening hemorrhage can occur with deficiencies in FXIII, α_2-antiplasmin, or von Willebrand Factor, all of which exhibit a normal PT/aPTT. Furthermore, FVIII and vWF levels are significantly increased during pregnancy and in response to physical stress or trauma. In such conditions, the aPTT may appear normal, thereby masking a true deficiency.

Furthermore, the aPTT may be markedly prolonged by a deficiency in FXII, which is not associated with bleeding, and the PT and/or aPTT may be prolonged by a lupus anticoagulant that increases the risk of thrombosis and not bleeding.

Finally, regardless of the cause, the degree to which the PT and/or aPTT is prolonged does not correlate with the severity of bleeding during invasive procedures, including neurosurgical procedures, such as intracranial pressure monitor placement.[56] Therefore, preoperative laboratory testing is not generally recommended for patients without a history of abnormal bleeding,[55] and an international normalized ratio value of less than 1.5, in the absence of bleeding, does not require attempted correction.[56]

Whole blood assays, including viscoelastic tests, may potentially improve the assessment of overall hemostatic function. However, these methods are similarly unable to assess important contributions from local tissue conditions and they cannot predict bleeding or thrombosis in unselected patients.

SUMMARY

The cascade model of coagulation is essential to interpreting the results of coagulation testing. However, neither this model, nor the PT and aPTT assays on which it was based, are capable of accurately reflecting the complexity of hemostasis in vivo.

Models of hemostasis have been improved by incorporating the contributions of different cell types and circulating inhibitors that combine to ensure the appropriate localization of coagulation reactions. However, these models are also incomplete, as they do not address the critical role of the fibrinolytic system, or the tissue-specific heterogeneity in the regulation of the hemostatic response.

The tissue-specific regulation of hemostasis relies on the differential expression of procoagulant and anticoagulant factors by endothelial cells at different sites throughout the vasculature. The brain, in particular, exhibits unique mechanisms of hemostatic regulation that favor increased activity of the FVIIa/TF pathway. This results in an unusually high degree of protection against hemorrhage, at the potential expense of increased thrombotic risk.

The specific regulation of these elements appears to be a distinct function of the blood-brain barrier, which relies on the interplay of endothelial cells, pericytes, and astrocytes in the cerebral microvasculature. As our understanding of this interplay increases, we will be better able to develop therapies that target or prevent cerebral vascular disease.

REFERENCES

1. Aird WC. Vascular bed-specific thrombosis. J Thromb Haemost 2007;5(Suppl 1):283–91.
2. Fisher MJ. Brain regulation of thrombosis and hemostasis: from theory to practice. Stroke 2013;44(11): 3275–85.
3. Mackman N. Tissue-specific hemostasis: role of tissue factor. J Thromb Haemost 2008;6(2):303–5.
4. Morawitz P. Die Chemie der Blutgerinnung. Ergeb Physiol 1905;4:307–422.
5. Quick AJ. The prothrombin time in hemophilia and in obstructive jaundice. J Biol Chem 1935;109:73–4.
6. Langdell RD, Wagner RH, Brinkhous KM. Effect of antihemophilic factor on one-stage clotting tests; a presumptive test for hemophilia and a simple one-stage antihemophilic factor assay procedure. J Lab Clin Med 1953;41(4):637–47.
7. Proctor RR, Rapaport SI. The partial thromboplastin time with kaolin. A simple screening test for first stage plasma clotting factor deficiencies. Am J Clin Pathol 1961;36:212–9.
8. Macfarlane RG. An enzyme cascade in the blood clotting mechanism, and its function as a biochemical amplifier. Nature 1964;202:498–9.
9. Davie EW, Ratnoff OD. Waterfall sequence for intrinsic blood clotting. Science 1964;145(3638): 1310–2.
10. Addison W. On the colourless corpuscles and on the molecules and cytoblasts in the blood. London Med Gaz 1842;30:144–8.
11. Virchow R. Gesammelte abhandlungen zur wissenschaftlichen medicin. Frankfurt (Germany): Medinger Sohn & Co; 1856.
12. Hoffman M, Monroe DM 3rd. A cell-based model of hemostasis. Thromb Haemost 2001;85(6):958–65.
13. Fleck RA, Rao LV, Rapaport SI, et al. Localization of human tissue factor antigen by immunostaining with monospecific, polyclonal anti-human tissue factor antibody. Thromb Res 1990;59(2):421–37.
14. Drake TA, Morrissey JH, Edgington TS. Selective cellular expression of tissue factor in human tissues. Implications for disorders of hemostasis and thrombosis. Am J Pathol 1989;134(5):1087–97.
15. Neuenschwander PF, Fiore MM, Morrissey JH. Factor VII autoactivation proceeds via interaction of distinct protease-cofactor and zymogen-cofactor complexes. Implications of a two-dimensional enzyme kinetic mechanism. J Biol Chem 1993; 268(29):21489–92.
16. Osterud B, Rapaport SI. Activation of factor IX by the reaction product of tissue factor and factor VII: additional pathway for initiating blood coagulation. Proc Natl Acad Sci U S A 1977;74(12): 5260–4.
17. Monkovic DD, Tracy PB. Functional characterization of human platelet-released factor V and its activation

by factor Xa and thrombin. J Biol Chem 1990; 265(28):17132–40.

18. Ayombil F, Abdalla S, Tracy PB, et al. Proteolysis of plasma-derived factor V following its endocytosis by megakaryocytes forms the platelet-derived factor V/Va pool. J Thromb Haemost 2013;11(8):1532–9.

19. Tracy PB, Rohrbach MS, Mann KG. Functional prothrombinase complex assembly on isolated monocytes and lymphocytes. J Biol Chem 1983;258(12): 7264–7.

20. Le DT, Borgs P, Toneff TW, et al. Hemostatic factors in rabbit limb lymph: relationship to mechanisms regulating extravascular coagulation. Am J Physiol 1998;274(3 Pt 2):H769–76.

21. Hoffman M, Colina CM, McDonald AG, et al. Tissue factor around dermal vessels has bound factor VII in the absence of injury. J Thromb Haemost 2007;5(7): 1403–8.

22. Hung DT, Vu TK, Wheaton VI, et al. Cloned platelet thrombin receptor is necessary for thrombin-induced platelet activation. J Clin Invest 1992; 89(4):1350–3.

23. Oliver JA, Monroe DM, Roberts HR, et al. Thrombin activates factor XI on activated platelets in the absence of factor XII. Arterioscler Thromb Vasc Biol 1999;19(1):170–7.

24. Ariens RA, Lai TS, Weisel JW, et al. Role of factor XIII in fibrin clot formation and effects of genetic polymorphisms. Blood 2002;100(3):743–54.

25. Olson ST, Richard B, Izaguirre G, et al. Molecular mechanisms of antithrombin-heparin regulation of blood clotting proteinases. A paradigm for understanding proteinase regulation by serpin family protein proteinase inhibitors. Biochimie 2010;92(11): 1587–96.

26. Patnaik MM, Moll S. Inherited antithrombin deficiency: a review. Haemophilia 2008;14(6):1229–39.

27. Wood JP, Ellery PE, Maroney SA, et al. Biology of tissue factor pathway inhibitor. Blood 2014;123(19): 2934–43.

28. Dahm A, Van Hylckama Vlieg A, Bendz B, et al. Low levels of tissue factor pathway inhibitor (TFPI) increase the risk of venous thrombosis. Blood 2003; 101(11):4387–92.

29. Winckers K, ten Cate H, Hackeng TM. The role of tissue factor pathway inhibitor in atherosclerosis and arterial thrombosis. Blood Rev 2013;27(3):119–32.

30. Lu G, Broze GJ Jr, Krishnaswamy S. Formation of factors IXa and Xa by the extrinsic pathway: differential regulation by tissue factor pathway inhibitor and antithrombin III. J Biol Chem 2004;279(17): 17241–9.

31. Camire RM, Kalafatis M, Simioni P, et al. Platelet-derived factor Va/Va Leiden cofactor activities are sustained on the surface of activated platelets despite the presence of activated protein C. Blood 1998;91(8):2818–29.

32. Moll S. Thrombophilia: clinical-practical aspects. J Thromb Thrombolysis 2015;39(3):367–78.

33. Cohen MJ, Call M, Nelson M, et al. Critical role of activated protein C in early coagulopathy and later organ failure, infection and death in trauma patients. Ann Surg 2012;255(2):379–85.

34. Bouwens EA, Stavenuiter F, Mosnier LO. Mechanisms of anticoagulant and cytoprotective actions of the protein C pathway. J Thromb Haemost 2013; 11(Suppl 1):242–53.

35. Erickson LA, Ginsberg MH, Loskutoff DJ. Detection and partial characterization of an inhibitor of plasminogen activator in human platelets. J Clin Invest 1984;74(4):1465–72.

36. Tjarnlund-Wolf A, Brogren H, Lo EH, et al. Plasminogen activator inhibitor-1 and thrombotic cerebrovascular diseases. Stroke 2012;43(10):2833–9.

37. Weiler-Guettler H, Christie PD, Beeler DL, et al. A targeted point mutation in thrombomodulin generates viable mice with a prethrombotic state. J Clin Invest 1998;101(9):1983–91.

38. Mackman N. Tissue-specific hemostasis in mice. Arterioscler Thromb Vasc Biol 2005;25(11):2273–81.

39. Vanassche T, Hirsh J, Eikelboom JW, et al. Organ-specific bleeding patterns of anticoagulant therapy: lessons from clinical trials. Thromb Haemost 2014; 112(5):918–23.

40. Kim JH, Kim JH, Park JA, et al. Blood-neural barrier: intercellular communication at glio-vascular interface. J Biochem Mol Biol 2006;39(4):339–45.

41. Liu S, Agalliu D, Yu C, et al. The role of pericytes in blood-brain barrier function and stroke. Curr Pharm Des 2012;18(25):3653–62.

42. Eddleston M, de la Torre JC, Oldstone MB, et al. Astrocytes are the primary source of tissue factor in the murine central nervous system. A role for astrocytes in cerebral hemostasis. J Clin Invest 1993;92(1):349–58.

43. Bouchard BA, Shatos MA, Tracy PB. Human brain pericytes differentially regulate expression of procoagulant enzyme complexes comprising the extrinsic pathway of blood coagulation. Arterioscler Thromb Vasc Biol 1997;17(1):1–9.

44. Jackson CM, Esnouf MP. Has the time arrived to replace the quick prothrombin time test for monitoring oral anticoagulant therapy? Clin Chem 2005; 51(3):483–5.

45. Hoffman M, Monroe DM. Tissue factor in brain is not saturated with factor VIIa: implications for factor VIIa dosing in intracerebral hemorrhage. Stroke 2009; 40(8):2882–4.

46. Bajaj MS, Kuppuswamy MN, Manepalli AN, et al. Transcriptional expression of tissue factor pathway inhibitor, thrombomodulin and von Willebrand factor in normal human tissues. Thromb Haemost 1999; 82(3):1047–52.

47. Xu Y, Slayter HS. Immunocytochemical localization of endogenous anti-thrombin III in the vasculature

of rat tissues reveals locations of anticoagulantly active heparan sulfate proteoglycans. J Histochem Cytochem 1994;42(10):1365–76.

48. Butros LJ, Bussel JB. Intracranial hemorrhage in immune thrombocytopenic purpura: a retrospective analysis. J Pediatr Hematol Oncol 2003;25(8):660–4.

49. Wong VL, Hofman FM, Ishii H, et al. Regional distribution of thrombomodulin in human brain. Brain Res 1991;556(1):1–5.

50. Yang F, Liu S, Wang SJ, et al. Tissue plasminogen activator expression and barrier properties of human brain microvascular endothelial cells. Cell Physiol Biochem 2011;28(4):631–8.

51. Laszik Z, Mitro A, Taylor FB Jr, et al. Human protein C receptor is present primarily on endothelium of large blood vessels: implications for the control of the protein C pathway. Circulation 1997;96(10): 3633–40.

52. Zlokovic BV, Griffin JH. Cytoprotective protein C pathways and implications for stroke and neurological disorders. Trends Neurosci 2011; 34(4):198–209.

53. Shatos MA, Orfeo T, Doherty JM, et al. Alpha-thrombin stimulates urokinase production and DNA synthesis in cultured human cerebral microvascular endothelial cells. Arterioscler Thromb Vasc Biol 1995;15(7):903–11.

54. Pannell R, Li S, Gurewich V. Fibrin-specific and effective clot lysis requires both plasminogen activators and for them to be in a sequential rather than simultaneous combination. J Thromb Thrombolysis 2017;44(2):210–5.

55. Chee YL, Crawford JC, Watson HG, et al. Guidelines on the assessment of bleeding risk prior to surgery or invasive procedures. British Committee for Standards in Haematology. Br J Haematol 2008;140(5): 496–504.

56. West KL, Adamson C, Hoffman M. Prophylactic correction of the international normalized ratio in neurosurgery: a brief review of a brief literature. J Neurosurg 2011;114(1):9–18.

Evaluation of Coagulation in the Neurosurgery Patient

George M. Rodgers, MD, PhD

KEYWORDS

- Coagulation testing • Hemostasis • Fibrinolysis • Viscoelastic assays • Thromboelastography
- Rotational elastometry • Traumatic brain injury

KEY POINTS

- Bleeding disorders can be categorized as platelet type or coagulation type.
- The bleeding time test is not a reliable assay to diagnose platelet-type bleeding disorders or to predict surgical bleeding.
- The gold standard assay for measuring platelet function is light transmission platelet aggregation.
- The prothrombin time and partial thromboplastin time are the 2 primary screening tests used to assess coagulation. These assays (and the International Normalized Ratio) predict bleeding and mortality in neurosurgical patients.
- Viscoelastic assays are useful in guiding transfusion therapy and diagnosing hyperfibrinolysis in neurosurgical patients. Their use in guiding treatment decisions is controversial.

OVERVIEW OF HEMOSTASIS

Achieving and maintaining adequate hemostasis is critical in management of neurosurgical patients. Even minor bleeding may have severe clinical consequences. This article reviews normal hemostatic mechanisms, summarizes traditional and emerging coagulation tests that are relevant for neurosurgical patients, reviews the clinical usefulness of standard and newer coagulation tests in neurosurgery practice with a focus on patients with traumatic brain injury (TBI), and provides an overview of common bleeding disorders and their laboratory evaluation.

Mechanisms of Normal Hemostasis

The prevention of excessive bleeding after vascular injury relies on normal hemostasis, which provides for balanced interactions between the vessel wall, coagulation proteins, and platelets.[1] After vascular injury, vascular constriction occurs in association with platelet aggregation and fibrin formation.

Normal hemostasis includes primary hemostasis, which involves platelet adhesion and aggregation, and secondary hemostasis, which involves thrombin generation and the formation of a fibrin mesh that reinforces the platelet thrombus. Defects in either hemostatic pathway may result in a bleeding disorder. After hemostasis has been achieved, blood vessel patency is restored by the fibrinolytic mechanism.

Excessive bleeding may result either from defects in primary hemostasis (platelet number or platelet function), defects in secondary hemostasis (coagulation protein deficiency), or excessive fibrinolysis.

Primary Hemostasis

In the absence of vascular injury, the normal vessel wall expresses antiplatelet and anticoagulant

Disclosures: None.
Division of Hematology and Hematologic Malignancies, University of Utah Health Sciences Center, 30 North 1900 East, Salt Lake City, UT 84132, USA
E-mail address: george.rodgers@hsc.utah.edu

Neurosurg Clin N Am 29 (2018) 485–492
https://doi.org/10.1016/j.nec.2018.06.001

activities that maintain blood in the fluid state and prevent activation of platelets and the coagulation mechanism.[2] However, with blood vessel injury, subendothelium is exposed that contains collagen fibrils, which induce binding of von Willebrand factor to platelets. Glycoprotein (GP) Ib is the platelet von Willebrand factor receptor required for platelet adhesion. Subsequent platelet activation leads to platelet aggregation, which is mediated by fibrinogen and its receptor, platelet GP IIbIIIa. Therefore, the defects in primary hemostasis that could lead to bleeding include deficiency of platelet GP 1b or GP IIbIIIa, deficiency of von Willebrand factor (von Willebrand disease), thrombocytopenia, or platelet dysfunction.[1]

Secondary Hemostasis

An effective clot requires fibrin consolidation (reinforcement) of the initial platelet thrombus; otherwise, delayed bleeding may occur. Secondary hemostasis involves thrombin generation and fibrin formation to provide this consolidation.

Typically, the blood coagulation mechanism is initiated by vessel trauma that exposes extravascular tissue factor to blood.[1] Tissue factor is present in the subendothelial matrix and fibroblasts; exposure of tissue factor to coagulation factor VII in blood initiates the coagulation pathway, leading to thrombin formation. The coagulation pathway is summarized in **Fig. 1**; it involves sequential enzymatic conversions of precursor coagulation zymogens to proteases that ultimately result in conversion of prothrombin to thrombin. Thrombin then activates platelets and converts soluble fibrinogen to an insoluble fibrin clot. Defects in secondary hemostasis that could result in bleeding include deficiency of or antibody to prothrombin (factor II), fibrinogen, and factors V, VII, VIII, IX, X, XI, and XIII.[1]

Fibrinolysis

After cessation of bleeding by formation of the hemostatic plug, repair of the blood vessel begins with lysis of the fibrin clot.[1] Endothelial cells of the vessel wall secrete tissue plasminogen activator (TPA); activation of plasminogen by TPA produces plasmin, a protease that induces clot lysis. Fibrinolysis is regulated by inhibitors to TPA (plasminogen activator inhibitor) and plasmin (α_2-antiplasmin). Defects in fibrinolysis that could result in bleeding include excessive secretion of TPA or deficiency of plasminogen activator inhibitor or α_2-antiplasmin.[1] **Fig. 2** summarizes hemostatic events that occur after vascular injury, including

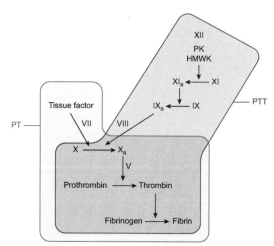

Fig. 1. The coagulation pathway and coagulation assays (prothrombin time [PT], partial thromboplastin time [PTT]) used to measure coagulation factor activities. The PT measures the tissue factor/factor VII pathway and common pathway (fibrinogen, prothrombin, factors V and X); this pathway is initiated in vivo with vascular injury when extravascular tissue factor interacts with factor VII to activate factor X. The PTT measures the common coagulation pathway plus 6 additional coagulation factors, namely, factor XII, PK, HMWK, factor VIII, factor IX, and factor XI. Factor XII, PK, and HMWK are necessary for in vitro coagulation, but not in vivo coagulation. The endpoint of both the PT and PTT assays is conversion of fibrinogen to fibrin. Factor XIII activity (not shown) is not measured by the PT or PTT assays. HMWK, high-molecular-weight kininogen; PK, prekallikrein; PT, prothrombin time; PTT, partial thromboplastin time.

platelet adhesion and aggregation, thrombin generation, and fibrin formation.

APPROACH TO THE BLEEDING PATIENT

Before laboratory testing, historical questions may provide useful information as to the type of bleeding disorder.[3] Asking about the duration of the bleeding tendency can aid in distinguishing inherited versus acquired bleeding disorders. Inquiring about a familial bleeding history can suggest if the bleeding disorder is transmitted in a dominant versus recessive manner. Asking whether bleeding is spontaneous versus requiring surgery or trauma can indicate if the bleeding disorder is severe or mild. The presence of petechial rash and small bruises suggest a platelet-type bleeding disorder, whereas large soft tissue hematomas, visceral bleeding, and hemarthrosis suggest a coagulation-type bleeding disorder. **Table 1** summarizes differences between platelet-type versus coagulation-type bleeding disorders.

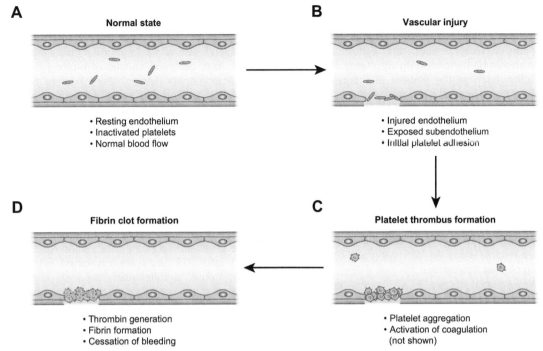

Fig. 2. Overview of platelet function and coagulation in response to vascular injury. (*A*) In the normal state, endothelium is intact, blood flow is normal, and platelets are in the resting state. (*B*) After vascular injury, the subendothelium is exposed, resulting in platelet adhesion, a process mediated by von Willebrand factor. (*C*) Platelet activation leads to platelet aggregation, a process mediated by fibrinogen. (*D*) The coagulation pathway is initiated, leading to thrombin generation, conversion of fibrinogen to fibrin, reinforcement of the platelet plug, and cessation of bleeding.

LABORATORY EVALUATION OF HEMOSTASIS
Assessing Platelets and Platelet Function

Routine platelet counts are obtained from the complete blood count that quantitates platelet number using an automated particle counter. Confirmation of the automated platelet count is easily performed by viewing the patient's peripheral blood smear.

The older medical literature supported the use of the template bleeding time test to measure in vitro platelet function. Physicians would order the test to screen for platelet dysfunction and to predict which patients might bleed with surgery or procedures. Unfortunately, although bleeding time is affected by platelet number and function, it is also affected by hematocrit, skin quality, testing technique, and other variables. More recent data indicate that there is no evidence that this test predicts bleeding[4,5] and there is no correlation between a skin template bleeding time and a visceral bleeding time in a given patient.[6] With regard to neurosurgery, an animal study found no relationship between the skin template bleeding time and a brain bleeding time.[7] Consensus guidelines from clinical laboratory

Table 1
Features of platelet-type versus coagulation-type bleeding

Characteristics	Platelet-Type Bleeding	Coagulation-Type Bleeding
Gender	Females > males	Males > females
Inheritance	Autosomal-dominant usually	X-linked recessive usually
Bleeding	Mucosal Small bruises Trivial cuts cause bleeding Bleeding is mild to moderate	Hemarthrosis Large bruises Trivial cuts do not cause bleeding Bleeding is moderate to severe

associations recommend that the bleeding time test not be performed.[8] If a patient is suspected of having a platelet-type bleeding disorder, tests for von Willebrand disease and platelet dysfunction should be performed. In vitro tests of platelet function such as the Platelet Function Analyzer (PFA)-100 (Siemens, Munich, Germany) may be more predictive than the bleeding time test; however, an expert committee of the International Society on Thrombosis and Hemostasis does not recommend the PFA-100 for routine clinical use, based on a lack of clinical outcome data.[9]

Despite numerous attempts to simplify measurement of platelet function, the gold standard test remains light transmission platelet aggregometry. Although the test is labor intensive and is not available on an emergent basis, it remains the most reliable assay for identifying and characterizing platelet dysfunction.[10]

Newer point-of-care (POC) assays have been developed to measure platelet function, such as the VerifyNow (Accriva, San Diego, CA). This system uses whole blood to measure platelet aggregation with fibrinogen-coated microparticles induced by platelet agonists. These assays can be used to identify potential bleeding risks in patients taking aspirin or to identify patients with thrombotic risk who are taking antiplatelet drugs.[11] The VerifyNow assay has been used in cardiac surgery and procedures.[12] However, a recent literature review of POC tests concluded that these assays were only of modest usefulness when used to predict clopidogrel resistance in cardiology patients.[11]

Assessing Coagulation

The prothrombin time (PT) and partial thromboplastin time (PTT) are the 2 primary screening tests used to assess the coagulation pathway. The PT assay measures the common pathway (fibrinogen, prothrombin, and factors V and X) and factor VII; a prolonged PT clotting time usually results from decreased levels of one or more of these clotting factors.[1] The International Normalized Ratio (INR) is a mathematical derivation term used to monitor PT results in patients on warfarin (Coumadin) anticoagulation. The INR is frequently used as a surrogate parameter for the PT assay.

The PTT assay measures the common pathway in addition to factors VIII, IX, XI, and XII; prekallikrein; and high-molecular-weight kininogen. Factor XII, prekallikrein, high-molecular-weight kininogen, when deficient, prolong the PTT test, but their deficiency is not associated with excessive bleeding. Thus, the clinically relevant coagulation factors measured by the PTT assay are the common pathway factors (fibrinogen, prothrombin, and factors V and X), and factors VIII, IX, and XI.[1] A prolonged PTT time usually results from decreased levels of one (or more) of these clotting factors; less common causes of prolonged PTT tests include antibodies or other inhibitors (heparin, argatroban, and direct oral anticoagulants).

It should be noted that neither the PT assay nor the PTT assay measure factor XIII activity.

How Do We Use the Prothrombin Time and Partial Thromboplastin Time Assays to Assess Bleeding Risk?

Because PT and PTT assays are widely available on a stat basis in virtually all hospitals and clinics, using them provides a rapid and efficient way to assess a patients' bleeding risk. When results of the PT and PTT tests are combined with the platelet count, a differential diagnosis can be generated that suggests additional laboratory testing to confirm a specific bleeding disorder. **Table 2** summarizes this approach. This approach assumes that a patient is bleeding for hemostatic reasons and not for structural reasons (lacerated blood vessel, arteriovenous malformation). Combining the results of this analysis with the patient's past medical history and medications usually leads to correct classification of the disorder being inherited or acquired, a disorder of primary hemostasis versus secondary hemostasis, and a relevant list of diagnostic possibilities to further evaluate.[1] The next section reviews some confirmatory coagulation tests useful in evaluation of bleeding disorders.

OTHER COAGULATION TESTS
Thrombin Time

This test measures the terminal step of coagulation, namely, the conversion of fibrinogen to fibrin. Abnormal thrombin time results may be due to heparin, low fibrinogen levels, an abnormal fibrinogen (dysfibrinogen), and elevated fibrin degradation products. The thrombin time assay is most commonly used to evaluate isolated prolonged PTT values for the presence of heparin.

Peripheral Blood Smear

A review of the patients' blood smear is helpful to confirm thrombocytopenia or thrombocytosis and to evaluate for possible causes of an abnormal platelet count.

Disseminated Intravascular Coagulation Panel

Disseminated intravascular coagulation (DIC) may occur in patients with TBI. The best single test to

Table 2
Differential diagnosis of hemostasis screening tests in patients with common bleeding disorders

PT	PTT	Platelet Count	Differential Diagnosis	Confirmatory Testing
↑	N	N	Factor VII deficiency: Liver disease Warfarin Vitamin K deficiency	Liver function tests
N	↑	N	Heparin Deficiency of: Factor VIII Factor IX Factor XI	Thrombin time, anti-factor X_a assay Factor assays
↑	↑	N	Liver disease Warfarin, superwarfarin Heparin Vitamin K deficiency	Liver function tests
↑	↑	↓	Liver disease DIC HIT	Liver function tests D-Dimer, fibrinogen Heparin-platelet factor 4 ELISA
N	N	N	Von Willebrand disease Platelet dysfunction Mild factor deficiency	Factor assays Platelet aggregation Factor assays
N	N	↓	Splenomegaly Decreased platelet production Increased platelet destruction	Abdominal imaging Hematology consult Hematology consult
N	N	↓	Myeloproliferative disorders Reactive thrombocytosis	Hematology consult An underlying disorder is present (trauma, infection, inflammation, cancer)

This table information assumes that structural bleeding has been excluded. Warfarin and superwarfarin (the active ingredient in rodenticides) can be confirmed by ordering specific drug tests. The PT and PTT are screening tests and may not detect patients with mild factor deficiency. Bleeding disorder patients with normal screening tests may require assay of all coagulation factors to achieve a diagnosis. HIT is usually a thrombotic disorder but may present with prolonged PT and PTT values with thrombocytopenia.

Abbreviations: ↓, decreased; ↑, increased; DIC, disseminated intravascular coagulation; ELISA, enzyme-linked immunosorbent assay; HIT, heparin-induced thrombocytopenia; N, normal; PT, prothrombin time; PTT, partial thromboplastin time.

diagnose DIC is a quantitative D-dimer assay. This sensitive assay measures activation of coagulation. Hospitalized patients or postoperative patients will have abnormal D-dimer assay results, but DIC is not diagnosed until the D-dimer value is greater than 8 μg/mL (8000 ng/mL).[13] Fibrinogen activity is another component of the DIC panel; many patients with DIC and bleeding will have low levels of fibrinogen that require replacement therapy with cryoprecipitate.

Specific Factor Assays

As summarized in **Table 2**, factor assays are useful in confirming many bleeding disorders, especially in patients with isolated prolonged PTT values. For this latter group of patients, if heparin use is excluded (with the thrombin time assay), assay of factors VIII, IX, and XI will identify the bleeding disorder.[1]

Mixing Study

Prolonged PT or PTT results are either due to factor deficiency or antibody (inhibitor) to a factor. The mixing test is a simple test to distinguish between these 2 possibilities. For example, if a patient has a prolonged PTT, mixing patient plasma with normal plasma will correct the prolonged PTT result if factor deficiency is present. If an antibody (or inhibitor such as heparin) is present, mixing patient plasma with normal plasma will not correct the prolonged PTT result.[3]

Platelet Aggregation Study

As mentioned elsewhere in this article, light transmission platelet aggregation is the gold standard test to assess platelet function. Unfortunately, it is affected by a long list of prescription and over-the-counter medications. It is ideally used to investigate outpatients suspected of a platelet function disorder before surgery. Importantly, patients need to abstain from aspirin, aspirin-containing medications, and other drugs that inhibit platelet function for up to 1 to 2 weeks before testing. It is impractical to use this assay to routinely evaluate hospitalized patients for platelet dysfunction.

EMERGING ASSAYS: POINT-OF-CARE VISCOELASTIC ANALYZERS

Three criticisms of standard hemostasis screening tests (PT, PTT, platelet count) are that these tests (1) take 1 to 2 hours to obtain results, (3) are artificial surrogate measures of hemostasis, that is, they are not cell-based assays, and (3) are not sensitive to hyperfibrinolysis. Because viscoelastic assays were developed to be POC tests, results are obtained in real time. By using whole blood, the viscoelastic tests aspire to measure hemostasis more completely because function of coagulation proteins and platelets are measured together. Two such assays are thromboelastography (TEG) and rotational elastometry (ROTEM).[14] In these assays, blood clots in a cuvette or cup in which a probe is suspended. The cup or probe is rotated, and the resulting viscoelastic forces between the 2 are recorded. Tracings from the analyzers indicate initial fibrin formation, clot strengthening, and clot stabilization. Clot lysis can also be recorded to measure excessive fibrinolysis.[14,15]

Many (but not all) studies have observed small but significant correlations between viscoelastic parameters and standard coagulation tests (platelet count, PTT). Details of these studies are discussed elsewhere in this article. Thus, transfusion protocols for blood products have been developed using these analyzers in the operative POC setting. Unfortunately, TEG is insensitive to the effects of antiplatelet drugs.[16]

The next section of this review discusses the clinical usefulness of standard coagulation testing and of the POC platelet function and viscoelastic assays, focusing on clinical trials involving patients with TBI.

CLINICAL USEFULNESS OF STANDARD COAGULATION TESTS IN NEUROSURGERY

Coagulopathy and bleeding occur frequently in patients with TBI. A Canadian study looked at the association of abnormal standard coagulation test results (INR, PTT, platelet count) in patients with severe TBI (Glasgow Coma Scale of ≤8).[17] Intracranial hemorrhage progressed in 80% of patients if any abnormal laboratory test occurred (INR of ≥1.3, PTT of >35 seconds, platelet count <100,000/μL) within the first 24 hours.[17]

A Chinese study evaluated predictive models to improve mortality prognosis in patients with TBI[18]; they found that INR values of greater than 1.25 and PTT values of greater than 36 seconds independently predicted hospital mortality. These authors also observed that these coagulation tests provided more useful information than standard admission variables such as age, pupillary reactivity, and Glasgow coma scale.[18] A literature metaanalysis investigated the usefulness of standard coagulation tests in diagnosing TBI and progressive bleeding.[19] A statistically significant positive correlation was observed between results of PT, INR, and D-dimer assays and progressive bleeding after TBI.[19]

The D-dimer assay was investigated in a Chinese study of TBI; patients with TBI who experienced progressive hemorrhage had higher D-dimer values than patients who did not have progressive hemorrhage.[20] A D-dimer cutoff value of 5 μg/mL was found to predict hemorrhage (odds ratio of approximately 12).[20]

An Australian study also investigated the relevance of standard coagulation tests such as the INR in patients with TBI.[21] A key finding was that normalization of the INR by blood products was independently associated with significantly lower mortality.[21] One conclusion from this study was that correction of TBI coagulopathy should occur as rapidly as possible. Their INR threshold for treatment is 1.3 or greater.[21]

In summary, numerous publications note the predictive power of routine coagulation tests such as the PT, INR, and D-dimer in patients with TBI. These tests not only predict bleeding, but also predict higher mortality, and their correction with treatment predicts lower mortality.

CLINICAL USEFULNESS OF POINT-OF-CARE PLATELET FUNCTION TESTING IN NEUROSURGICAL PATIENTS

As summarized, POC platelet function assays such as the VerifyNow device have been found to be of limited usefulness in the cardiology setting.[11] Mixed results also exist for these POC tests in the neurosurgical setting. For example, 1 study reported that the VerifyNow method was useful in identifying a subset of patients with TBI with occult platelet dysfunction.[22] In contrast, POC platelet function assays have not been found to be clinically useful in the neurointerventional setting (stenting). A study compared light transmission platelet aggregation, VerifyNow, and the Multiplate analyzer to assess platelet function in patients on clopidogrel undergoing neurovascular stenting; light transmission platelet aggregation was the best method to predict thrombotic complications.[23] The POC assays were less useful in predicting clinical outcomes.[23] Another neurointerventional study found similar results; using the VerifyNow test did not change the clinical outcomes.[24]

The VerifyNow test was also investigated in a retrospective study to predict bleeding and thrombosis in cerebral aneurysm patients treated with the Pipeline Embolization Device (Medtronic, Minneapolis, MN).[25] A preprocedure P2Y12 reaction unit value of less than 60 or greater than 240 independently predicted major perioperative hemostatic complications.[25]

The status of POC platelet function testing in neurosurgery patients can best be described as evolving. Although the POC viscoelastic tests (TEG, ROTEM, discussed elsewhere in this article) have significant usefulness in guiding transfusion therapy, there is no well-defined usefulness of the POC platelet function tests in neurosurgery patients. Randomized trials are needed using these assays to address issues such as standardization and appropriate laboratory cutoff values.[11]

CLINICAL USEFULNESS OF VISCOELASTIC TESTS IN NEUROSURGERY

The primary use of TEG and ROTEM is to guide transfusion therapy more quickly than standard coagulation assays.[14] Another advantage of viscoelastic tests over standard coagulation tests in neurosurgery is to rapidly identify hyperfibrinolysis in patients with TBI.[26] Hyperfibrinolysis can be associated with substantial mortality,[27] and identification of hyperfibrinolysis would lead to prompt treatment with antifibrinolytic therapy such as tranexamic acid.

A prospective trial evaluated the association between coagulopathy and mortality in patients with TBI.[28] These authors looked at standard coagulation tests and TEG. Higher mortality was seen in patients identified as hypocoagulable by TEG as well as in patients with abnormal PTT values or a low fibrinogen.[28]

A recent prospective study compared standard coagulation tests versus ROTEM parameters in patients undergoing emergent neurosurgery.[29] Coagulopathy was identified by standard tests in 35% of patients. There was a strong correlation between the 2 comparators. Both methods predicted the need for major red cell transfusion. These results validate previous studies that demonstrated correlations between standard coagulation testing and viscoelastic tests and confirm the predictive usefulness of viscoelastic tests to guide transfusion therapy.

Despite numerous publications on viscoelastic assays in the neurosurgery setting, large clinical trials demonstrating these tests improve clinical outcomes are lacking.[14,26] Some investigators have found that viscoelastic assays are not clinically useful in the management of patients with TBI.[30]

SUMMARY

Identifying patients at high risk of bleeding and preventing bleeding are key principles of caring for neurosurgery patients. We reviewed the role of standard coagulation tests and the new POC hemostasis tests in neurosurgery, with a focus on data in patients with TBI. Standard coagulation tests (PT, INR, PTT, D-dimer, platelet count) have been shown to be clinically useful in managing patients with TBI, but these tests have limitations. POC tests for platelet function and overall hemostasis (viscoelastic assays) have been developed, which successfully address laboratory result turnaround time concerns; however, these POC tests still have shortcomings.

There is a paucity of data for evaluating POC platelet function assays in the neurosurgery setting. More data exist for the viscoelastic tests (TEG, ROTEM), but advantages of these assays over standard coagulation assays seems to be limited. The uncertainty of using the viscoelastic assays is emphasized by a 2015 Cochrane Database systematic review on TEG and ROTEM use in trauma patients with coagulopathy and bleeding that concluded "these tests should only be used for research."[31] Although we have cited studies in neurosurgery patients published since the 2015 review, the number of recent studies is small.

Stronger data support the use of TEG and ROTEM in transfusion management of patients, but other patient care areas require additional studies, such as whether abnormal viscoelastic assay results should routinely lead to treatment interventions. Studies using viscoelastic assays in neurosurgery patients to determine treatment and measuring outcomes would provide useful information about the ultimate clinical usefulness of these tests.

REFERENCES

1. Rodgers GM. Coagulation and platelet plug formation. In: Hamilton MG, Golfinos JG, Pineo GF, et al, editors. Handbook of bleeding and coagulation for neurosurgery. New York: Thieme; 2015. p. 17–25.
2. Rodgers GM. Hemostatic properties of normal and perturbed vascular cells. FASEB J 1988;2:116–23.
3. Rudrapatna VK, Rodgers GM. Preoperative coagulation assessment for the neurosurgical patient. In:

Hamilton MG, Golfinos JG, Pineo GF, et al, editors. Handbook of bleeding and coagulation for neurosurgery. New York: Thieme; 2015. p. 26–37.

4. Lind SE. The Bleeding time does not predict surgical bleeding. Blood 1991;77:2547–52.

5. Lehman CM, Blaylock RC, Alexander DP, et al. Discontinuation of the bleeding time test without detectable adverse clinical impact. Clin Chem 2001;47:1204–11.

6. O'Laughlin JC, Hoftiezer JW, Mahoney JP, et al. Does aspirin prolong bleeding from gastric biopsies in man? Gastrointest Endosc 1981;27:1–5.

7. MacDonald JD, Remington BJ, Rodgers GM. The skin bleeding time test as a predictor of brain bleeding time in a rat model. Thromb Res 1994;76:535–40.

8. Peterson P, Hayes TE, Arkin CF, et al. The preoperative bleeding time test lacks clinical benefit: College of American Pathologists and American Society of Clinical Pathologists Position Article. Arch Surg 1998;133:134–9.

9. Hayward CP, Harrison P, Cattaneo M, et al. Platelet function analyzer (PFA)-100 closure time in the evaluation of platelet disorders and platelet function. J Thromb Haemost 2006;4:312–9.

10. Rodgers GM, Lehman CM. The diagnostic approach to the bleeding disorders. In: Greer JP, Arber DA, Glader B, et al, editors. Wintrobe's clinical hematology. Philadelphia: Lippincott Williams & Wilkins; 2014. p. 1043–57.

11. Le Quellec S, Bordet J-C, Negrier C, et al. Comparison of current platelet functional tests for the assessment of aspirin and clopidogrel response. Thromb Haemost 2016;116:638–50.

12. Welsh KJ, Dasgupta A, Nguyen AN, et al. Utility of VerifyNow™ for point-of-care identification of an aspirin effect prior to emergency cardiac surgery. Ann Clin Lab Sci 2015;45:377–81.

13. Lehman CM, Wilson LW, Rodgers GM. Analytic validation and clinical evaluation of the STA LIATEST immunoturbidometric D-dimer assay for the diagnosis of disseminated intravascular coagulation. Am J Clin Pathol 2004;122:178–84.

14. Hans GA, Besser MW. The place of viscoelastic testing in clinical practice. Br J Haematol 2016; 173:37–48.

15. Kvint S, Schuster J, Kumar MA. Neurosurgical applications of viscoelastic hemostatic assays. Neurosurg Focus 2017;43(5):E9.

16. Mylotte D, Foley D, Kenny D. Platelet function testing: methods of assessment and clinical utility. Cardiovasc Hematol Agents Med Chem 2011;9:14–24.

17. Allard CB, Scarpelini S, Rhind SG, et al. Abnormal coagulation tests are associated with progression of traumatic intracranial hemorrhage. J Trauma 2009;67:959–67.

18. Yuan Q, Yu J, Wu X, et al. Prognostic value of coagulation tests for in-hospital mortality in patients with traumatic brain injury. Scand J Trauma Resusc Emerg Med 2018;26:3.

19. Zhang D, Gong S, Jin H, et al. Coagulation parameters and risk of progressive hemorrhagic injury after traumatic brain injury: a systematic review and meta-analysis. Biomed Res Int 2015;2015:261825.

20. Tian HL, Chen H, Wu BS, et al. D-dimer as a predictor of progressive hemorrhagic injury in patients with traumatic brain injury: analysis of 194 cases. Neurosurg Rev 2010;33:359–65.

21. Epstein DS, Mitra B, Cameron PA, et al. Normalization of coagulopathy is associated with improved outcome after isolated traumatic brain injury. J Clin Neurosci 2016;29:64–9.

22. Gozal YM, Carroll CP, Krueger BM, et al. Point-of-care testing in the acute management of traumatic brain injury: identifying the coagulopathic patient. Surg Neurol Int 2017;8:48.

23. Flechtenmacher N, Kammerer F, Dittmer R, et al. Clopidogrel resistance in neurovascular stenting: correlations between light transmission aggregometry, VerifyNow™, and the Multiplate. AJNR Am J Neuroradiol 2015;36:1953–8.

24. Kass-Hout T, Alderaz YJ, Amuluru K, et al. Neurointerventional stenting and antiplatelet function testing: to do or not to do? Interv Neurol 2015;3:184–9.

25. Delgado JE, Crandall BM, Scholz JM, et al. Pre-procedure P2Y12 reaction units value predicts perioperative thromboembolic and hemorrhagic complications in patients with cerebral aneurysms treated with the Pipeline Embolization Device. J Neurointerv Surg 2013;5:iii3–10.

26. Beynon C, Wessels L, Unterberg AW. Point-of-care testing in neurosurgery. Semin Thromb Hemost 2017;43:416–22.

27. Schochl H, Frietsch T, Pavelka M, et al. Hyperfibrinolysis after major trauma: differential diagnosis of lysis patterns and prognostic value of thrombelastometry. J Trauma 2009;67:125–31.

28. Kunio NR, Differding JA, Watson KM, et al. Thromboelastography-identified coagulopathy is associated with increased morbidity and mortality after traumatic brain injury. Am J Surg 2012;203:584–8.

29. Ellenberger C, Garofano N, Barcelos G, et al. Assessment of haemostasis in patients undergoing emergent neurosurgery by rotational elastometry and standard coagulation tests: a prospective observational study. BMC Anesthesiol 2017;17:146.

30. Rao AJ, Laurie A, Hilliard C, et al. The utility of thromboelastography for predicting the risk of progression of intracranial hemorrhage in traumatic brain injury patients [abstract]. Clin Neurosurg 2016;63:173–4.

31. Hunt H, Stanworth S, Curry N, et al. Thromboelastography (TEG) and rotational thromboelastometry (ROTEM) for trauma-induced coagulopathy in adult trauma patients with bleeding. Cochrane Database Syst Rev 2015;(2):CD010438.

Genetics of Hypercoagulable and Hypocoagulable States

Daulath Singh, MD[a],*, Arjun Natarajan, MBBS, MD[b],
Sucha Nand, MD[a], Hanh P. Mai, DO[a]

KEYWORDS

- Factor V Leiden • Prothrombin gene mutation • Protein C and S deficiencies
- Antithrombin deficiency • Antiphospholipid syndrome • von Willebrand disease • Hemophilia

KEY POINTS

- Hemostasis is a tightly regulated process, and a delicate equilibrium exists between prothrombotic and antithrombotic factors.
- Hypercoagulable states can be acquired or inherited.
- Inherited thrombophilia can be inherited in a heterozygous or homozygous fashion with varying degrees of penetrance.
- Antiphospholipid syndrome is associated with significant venous and arterial thrombosis as well as obstetric complications.
- Inherited bleeding disorders include von Willebrand disease and hemophilia.

Under physiologic conditions, equilibrium exists between thrombotic and antithrombotic mechanisms. Primary hemostasis involves the interaction of endothelial cells, von Willebrand factor (VWF), and platelets to form a temporary platelet plug. Secondary hemostasis, also known as the coagulation cascade, involves a series of enzymatic reactions culminating in the formation of a stable fibrin clot (**Fig. 1**).[1,2] Venous stasis, hypercoagulability (either inherited or acquired causes), and vascular injury are predisposing risk factors for thrombosis.[3] Protein C, S, and antithrombin (AT) are natural anticoagulants of the coagulation cascade. Thrombin converts protein C to activated protein C (APC), which, in combination with protein S inactivates factors Va and VIIIa, providing a negative feedback loop to effectively limit thrombin production. AT binds to and inactivates thrombin, factor Xa, as well as other clotting factors.

It has been known for centuries that inherited defects in the coagulation system can lead to bleeding diatheses. However, the counterargument, which is inherited defects leading to the increased risk of pathologic thrombosis, has been elucidated only in the last few decades.[2,4] Over the last century, research has been performed to identify the genetic causes of thrombophilia. A hereditary thrombophilia results when there is a deficiency in a clotting protein, which can be inherited in a homozygous or heterozygous fashion. Homozygosity is the loss of 2 gene copies, resulting in the total loss of the protein product. Heterozygosity refers to the loss of one gene copy, where there is still some functional product present. The severity of the clinical

Disclosure: The authors have nothing to disclose.
[a] Department of Hematology and Oncology, Loyola University Medical Center, 2160 South First Avenue, Maywood, IL 60153, USA; [b] Department of Internal Medicine, Advocate Illinois Masonic Medical Center, 533 West Barry Avenue, Unit 7K, Chicago, IL 60657, USA
* Corresponding author.
E-mail address: Daulath.singh@lumc.edu

Neurosurg Clin N Am 29 (2018) 493–501
https://doi.org/10.1016/j.nec.2018.06.002

INTRINSIC

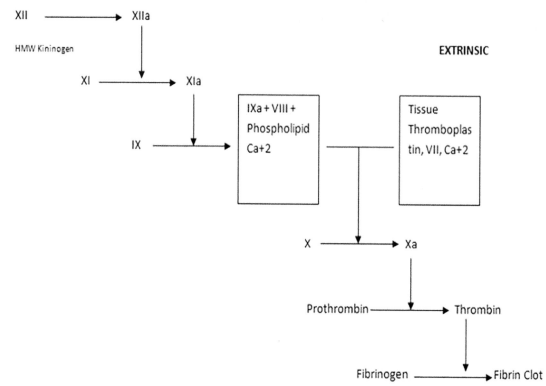

Fig. 1. Extrinsic and intrinsic pathways of coagulation. HMW, high molecular weight. (*From* Aneeque M. Coagulation cascade. Available at: https://www.slideshare.net/muhammadakhan754365/coagulation-cascade-dr-m-aneeque; with permission. Accessed March 16, 2018.)

phenotype or thrombotic risk depends on the homozygous or heterozygous state.[1,5] The common causes of inherited thrombophilia include factor V Leiden (FVL), prothrombin gene mutation, protein C, protein S, and AT deficiencies.

INHERITED AND ACQUIRED HYPERCOAGULABLE STATES
Factor V Leiden or Activated Protein C Resistance

APC is a potent inhibitor of the coagulation system. It cleaves the activated forms of factors V and VIII. In 1993, Dahlback and colleagues discovered that patients with resistance to APC developed clinical thrombosis, and the mode of inheritance appeared to be autosomal dominant. In 1994, Bertina and colleagues described a single point mutation in the factor V gene resulting in susceptibility of inactivation by APC. Factor V gene has been mapped to chromosome 1 (1q21-25) and is closely linked to the AT gene.[6] The term "activated protein C resistance" was developed because of the observation that APC in patients' plasma failed to prolong the partial thromboplastin

time (PTT). A substitution mutation at nucleotide 1691 results in the replacement of arginine by glutamine. This gene product, called factor V Leiden (FVL), also known as factor V Q506 or Arg506Gln, is named after the city in the Netherlands where it was first identified. FVL is a variant of the normal gene and is not susceptible to cleavage at position 506 by APC (**Fig. 2**). Consequently, more factor Va is available within the prothrombinase complex, thereby increasing the generation of thrombin. FVL is the most common cause of heritable thrombophilia.[1,2,7] The prevalence of heterozygous FVL is 3% to 8% in the Caucasian population and 1.2% in African Americans. Homozygous FVL occurs in 1 in 500 to 1600 Caucasians.[2] Based on published case control studies, there is a 5- to 10-fold increase in thrombosis risk in heterozygous carriers and approximately 80-fold increase in thrombosis risk for homozygous carriers.[7] A study of 306 members from 50 Swedish families found that 40% of homozygous individuals had an episode of venous thrombosis by age 33, compared with 20% of heterozygous individuals, and 8% of normal.[1,6,7] The risk of recurrent venous thromboembolism (VTE)

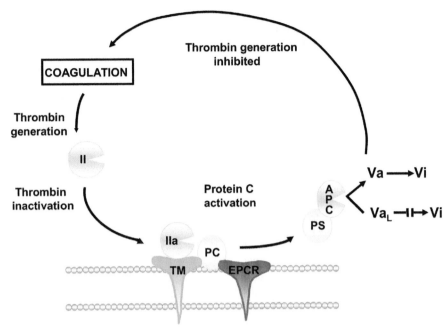

Fig. 2. The protein C/protein S pathway is complementary to the AT-III pathway. When thrombin binds to thrombomodulin, thrombin undergoes a conformational change and no longer clots fibrinogen or activates platelets. However, it acquires the ability to activate protein C in plasma. Protein S serves as a cofactor for APC. APC degrades activated factor V and FVIII, the 2 cofactors in the clotting cascade. (*From* Anderson JAM, Weitz JI. Hypercoagulable states. Clin Chest Med 2010;31:662; with permission.)

in heterozygous FVL is modestly increased. The risk of recurrence in homozygous carriers is estimated to be 2.65-fold. A meta-analysis demonstrated the risk of arterial thromboembolic events is 1.21-fold greater in FVL carriers compared with the normal population.[2] Diagnosis involves an activated partial thromboplastin time–based screening assay involving APC resistance. An abnormal APC resistance test is then confirmed by gene sequencing with polymerase chain reaction (PCR).[2]

Prothrombin Gene Mutation

Prothrombin (factor II) is the precursor to thrombin and has procoagulant, anticoagulant, and antifibrinolytic activities. In 1996, Poort and colleagues first described a single amino acid genetic change in the 3′ untranslated region of the gene that codes for prothrombin. An observational study of 28 families from the Netherlands with known VTE identified a substitution of guanine to adenine at nucleotide 20210 in the 3′ untranslated region of the prothrombin gene. Individuals with the G20210A allele have an odds ratio of 2.8 of developing venous thrombosis. Both elevated prothrombin and the presence of the allele are risk factors for thrombosis. Heterozygous carriers have a 30% higher plasma prothrombin level than normal individuals. The highest prevalence

for heterozygous prothrombin mutation, which varies from 0.7% to 6.5%, is reported in Spain. This mutation is rare in non-Caucasian populations.[1,7] Heterozygotes have a 2- to 5-fold increase in thrombosis risk compared with the normal population. Prothrombin mutation can be coinherited with another thrombophilia, such as FVL, protein C, S, or AT deficiencies.[2,7] This point mutation is the second most common known inherited risk factor for venous thrombosis, after FVL. It is inherited in an autosomal dominant fashion. Homozygosity occurs in approximately 1 in 4000 individuals of Caucasian heritage. Diagnosis is based on genetic testing or PCR. The risk for first VTE is similar to FVL. Heterozygosity for the prothrombin mutation confers a 3-fold increased risk for first-time VTE. The exact risk for recurrent VTE is unknown. A meta-analysis has failed to demonstrate a meaningful association between having prothrombin mutation and increased risk of arterial thromboembolism.[1,2]

Protein C Deficiency

Protein C is a vitamin K–dependent protein, which is converted during the coagulation process to APC. Inherited protein C deficiency was first described in 1981 as a cause of thromboembolism. The gene for protein C is located on chromosome 2 (2q13-14) and appears to be closely linked to the gene that codes for factor IX (FIX). More than 160 mutations involving the protein C gene have been described. More than half of the known mutations are either missense or nonsense mutations.[1] Two types of deficiency exist: type I is a quantitative deficiency, and type II is a qualitative deficiency characterized by a low activity but normal antigen level. Regarding the risk of thrombosis, the distinction between the 2 subtypes is not clinically significant. It is inherited in an autosomal dominant fashion. Prevalence in the general population is 1 in 500 to 600. Homozygous or double heterozygous protein C deficiency occurs in 1 per 1 million pregnancies. It is recommended to obtain both protein C activity and antigen level to diagnose. The risk of first VTE is increased 4- to 7-fold. The annual incidence of a first VTE is 1.52% compared with 0.1% in the general population. Protein C deficiency is modestly associated with a risk of recurrent VTE. The risk of arterial thrombosis has not been established in protein C deficiency.[2] Patients with protein C deficiency initiated on Coumadin are at risk for Coumadin-induced skin necrosis because of a transient hypercoagulable state induced by Coumadin with depletion of protein C and S in the setting of already low protein C level.[2]

Protein S Deficiency

Protein S exists in 2 states: free or as a complex with a transport protein called C4b-binding protein. In its free form, it functions as a natural anticoagulant, by being a cofactor for APC to inactive factor Va and factor VIIIa. This entity was first described in 1984. There are 2 homologous genes for protein S: PROS1 and PROS2, both of which are mapped to chromosome 3. To date, more than 131 different mutations have been identified. It is inherited in an autosomal dominant fashion. Homozygous or double heterozygous mutations can lead to early onset of VTE or severe neonatal purpura fulminans. Three types of deficiency exist: type I, type II, and type III. These 3 phenotypes have been described based on the total protein S antigen concentration, free protein S concentration, and protein S functional activity. The true prevalence of protein S deficiency is unknown and may range between 1 in 800 and 1 in 3000. Measuring both free protein S antigen and activity is recommended to make an accurate diagnosis. It is important to realize that there are multiple causes of acquired protein S deficiency, such as high factor VIII (FVIII) levels, presence of FVL mutation, lupus anticoagulant (LA), use of oral contraceptive agents, pregnancy, liver disease, nephrotic syndrome, disseminated intravascular coagulation, and use of vitamin K antagonists.[1,2,7]

Antithrombin Deficiency

Published literature in the 1960s reported an association between the development of VTE and reduced levels of AT. Since this discovery, 250 different mutations of AT deficiency have been reported. AT is a single-chain glycoprotein made in the liver. It belongs to the serine protease inhibitor superfamily and inactivates thrombin, factors Xa, IXa, XIa, and XIIa. AT deficiency is usually inherited in an autosomal dominant fashion. Four clinical subtypes have been described: type I deficiency is characterized by a reduced synthesis of normal protease inhibitor molecules, leading to a reduction in antigenic and functional activity of plasma AT. In the heterozygous state, the level is approximately 50% of normal. Type II deficiency is characterized by a discrete molecular defect within the protein. It is caused by point mutations causing single amino acid substitutions leading to a dysfunctional protein.[4,8] Type II can be further subdivided into 3 subtypes: abnormalities in the reactive site, heparin binding site, and those with effects on both heparin binding and protease inhibition. The AT-heparin cofactor activity is approximately 50% of normal AT activity in affected individuals.[1,8] Approximately 50% of selected AT-deficient patients develop thrombosis before the age of 40. About 50% of thrombotic events are idiopathic. The incidence of pregnancy-related thrombosis in AT-deficient women is greater than that of either protein C or S–deficient women.[2,7] Most affected patients are heterozygotes, with AT levels between 40% and 70% of normal, and homozygotes are rare.[4]

Antiphospholipid Syndrome

Antiphospholipid syndrome (APS) is defined as thrombosis and adverse obstetric events. APS is a common cause of acquired thrombophilia, which is remarkable for its association to both venous and arterial thromboembolism.[9] It is understood that the cause of thrombophilia is from antiphospholipid antibodies (aPLs), but the mechanism by which this occurs is only partially understood. The chief antigenic targets for these aPLs appear to be phospholipid binding plasma proteins, such as beta-2-glycoprotein 1 (B2GP1) and prothrombin.[10] B2GP1 is a plasma protein that is necessary for the binding of anticardiolipin (aCL) to solid phase phospholipids. The human B2GP1 gene is localized to chromosome 17q23. There are 4 major polymorphisms identified: Ser/Asn 88, Leu/Val 247, Cys/Gly 306, and Trp/Ser 316.[10] Genetic factors are thought to play a role in APS suscepti-bility. There have been reports of HLA class II al-leles, especially for DR and DQ antigens in patients with aPLs, including conventional aCL and/or anti-B2GP1 antibodies.[10] The 247 Val/Leu polymorphism can affect the conformational change of B2GP1 and exposure of aCL epitopes. The above polymorphism correlates with anti-B2GP1 production in patients with primary APS and may be important for B2GP1 antigenicity.[11] There also appears to be a correlation between Signal transducers and activators of transcription 4 single nucleotide polymorphism and APS, which was enhanced not only in patients with systemic lupus erythematosus (SLE) but also in those with primary APS, indicating a possible genetic associ-ation between SLE and APS.[12] It is particularly difficult to predict risk of first thrombosis in asymp-tomatic aPL carriers. LA positivity is a stronger risk factor for both arterial and venous thrombosis than aCL.[13] Immunoglobulin G anti-B2GP1 domain 1 antibodies are more strongly associated with thrombosis and obstetric morbidity compared with antibodies to other regions of the protein.[14] Patients with LA and anti-B2GP1 have a signifi-cantly increased risk for thrombosis based on data from the Warfarin in Antiphospholipid Syn-drome study.[15] It has also been shown that triple positivity for aCL, LA, and anti-B2GP1 has a higher risk of thrombosis.[16]

SPECIFIC INHERITED HYPOCOAGULABLE (BLEEDING) STATES
von Willebrand Disease

von Willebrand disease (VWD) is the most com-mon inherited bleeding disorder. It is either inherited in an autosomal dominant or autosomal recessive pattern.[17] In population-based studies, prevalence was estimated to be as high as 0.6% to 1.3%.[18,19]

VWF, a multimeric glycoprotein located on the short arm of chromosome 12, is synthesized by endothelial cells and megakaryocytes that mediate platelet adhesion/aggregation and stabi-lize FVIII in the circulation.[20–23]

VWD is subdivided into types 1, 2, and 3.[24] Type 1, accounting for 70% to 80% of cases, is charac-terized by a quantitative deficiency of VWF. Type 2, representing 20% of cases, is caused by a dysfunctional VWF, resulting in a normal or reduced VWF antigen concentration but a large reduction in VWF function. Type 2 is further subdi-vided based on specific phenotypic characteris-tics into 2A, 2B, 2M, and 2N. Type 3 is rare (<5% of cases), is the most severe form, and is caused by the absence of circulating VWF (**Table 1**).[25]

Most (~70%) mutations in type 1 VWD are missense mutations located in the VWF coding sequence, with splice site, transcription, small de-letions, small duplications, and nonsense muta-tions each representing less than 10% of the mutations found.[26] The most frequently reported genetic variation (10%–20% of index cases) iden-tified in all studies was a missense mutation result-ing in an amino acid substitution of tyrosine to cysteine at codon 1584 (Y1584C).[27] Defects in the VWF promoter have also been associated with type 1 VWD.[28] The typical inheritance pattern for type 1 VWD is autosomal dominant, and type 1 disease often shows variable expression and incomplete penetrance.

Type 2A VWD results from mutations that cause a defect in VWF activity through disruption of high-molecular-weight multimer (HMWM) formation. In-heritance follows an autosomal dominant pattern. Most mutations identified in type 2A VWD patients are missense and located in the A2 domain (56.7%), whereas 23.9% are in D′ and CK do-mains, and the remaining, 19.4%, are located in the A1 domain.[29] Type 2A VWD has been associ-ated with more than 50 different missense muta-tions that result in 2 types of pathogenetic mechanisms: either aberrant VWF dimer or multi-mer biosynthesis (group I mutations) or the synthe-sis of a protein with enhanced susceptibility to A disintegrin-like and metalloprotease with thrombo-spondin type 1 results (ADAMTS13)-mediated proteolysis (group II mutations).[30,31]

Type 2B VWD represents a gain-of-function defect in which VWF has an increased affinity for platelet GPIb. This results in clearance of VWF-platelet complexes, loss of HMWM, and, frequently, thrombocytopenia. Inheritance follows an autosomal dominant pattern.[17] Heterozygous mutations that cause VWD type 2B cluster within or near VWF domain A1 (coded by exon 28).[32]

Type 2M VWD is characterized by a defect in the ability of VWF to bind platelet GPIb and thus a decrease in VWF:RCo/VWF:Ag ratio, but with a normal multimer distribution. Inheritance follows an autosomal dominant pattern.[17] Causative mu-tations have been localized to the platelet GPIb binding site, in the A1 domain of VWF.[33,34]

Type 2N VWD results from defects in the ability of VWF to bind FVIII. Type 2N VWD results when 2 mutations in the FVIII binding region are present, one on each allele. It is also possible to have a 2N phenotype resulting from the presence of one type 2N mutation and one type 1 VWF mutation, typically resulting in low VWF or a null allele. There-fore, the inheritance pattern is autosomal reces-sive.[17] In contrast to type 1, the phenotype in type 2 disease is usually fully penetrant.[25]

Table 1
General characteristics of hemophilia A, B, and von Willebrand disease subtypes

Disorder	Prevalence	Mechanism	Variant Location by Protein Domain	Variant Location by Exon	Variant Types	Inheritance Pattern
HA	1/5000 males	Quantitative and qualitative FVIII deficiency	*F8* whole gene	1–26	Point mutations, insertions, deletions, inversions	X-linked recessive
HB	1/30,000 males	Quantitative and qualitative FIX deficiency	*F9* whole gene	1–8	Point mutations, insertions, deletions	X-linked recessive
Type 1 VWD	65%–80%	Partial VWF deficiency (VWF:Ag 0.05–0.5 U/mL)	*VWF* whole gene, external loci?	1–52, promoter	Point mutations, insertions, deletions	Autosomal dominant, occasional recessive, or codominant
Type 1C VWD	~15% of type 1	Accelerated VWF clearance from plasma	*VWF* D'D3, D4	18–27, 33–38	Missense variants	Autosomal dominant
Type 2A VWD	10%–20%	Impaired multimerization	*VWF* propeptide, D'D3, A1, CK	2–28, 51, 52	Missense variants	Autosomal dominant
Type 2B VWD	5%–10%	Gain-of-function binding to platelet GPIb	*VWF* A1	28	Missense variants	Autosomal dominant
Type 2M VWD	3%–5%	Impaired platelet GPIb or collagen binding	VWF A1, A2, A3	28–32	Missense variants	Autosomal dominant
Type 2N VWD	2%–5%	Decreased FVIII binding to VWF	*VWF* D'D3, propeptide cleavage site (2N), whole gene (null)	17–27 (2N) whole gene (null variant)	Missense variants, null variants (compound heterozygous)	Autosomal recessive homozygous, compound heterozygous
Type 3 VWD	1/1,000,000	Severe VWF deficiency (VWF:Ag <0.05 U/mL)	*VWF* whole gene	1–52	Point mutations, insertions, deletions	Autosomal recessive, codominant

From Swystun LL, James PD. Genetic diagnosis in hemophilia and von Willebrand disease. Blood Rev 2017;31:48; with permission.

Type 3 VWD presents with undetectable VWF protein. Inheritance is autosomal recessive, although parents of type 3 VWD patients may or may not be symptomatic. Type 3 VWD is due to disruption of expression from both VWF alleles, typically through either point mutations (missense or null) or deletions involving the *VWF* gene. In 80% of patients with type 3 VWD, the genetic defects in the *VWF* gene are null alleles, explaining the complete absence of VWF.[35,36] The most common deletion found to date is a deletion of exons 4 to 5.[37] Missense alterations comprise only approximately 15% of mutations in type 3 VWD.[38]

Hemophilia

Hemophilia is a genetic disease caused by mutation of one of the genes for coagulation proteins. The term usually refers to either hemophilia A (HA), indicating FVIII deficiency, or hemophilia B (HB), indicating FIX deficiency.[39] The genes encoding FVIII and FIX are on the long arm of the X chromosome. HA and HB are the only hereditary clotting diseases inherited in a sex-linked recessive pattern. Their severity is currently classified based on the plasma levels of FVIII or FIX activity: severe (<1%), moderate (1%–5%), and mild (>5% to <40%) of normal activity.[40]

HA is caused by dysfunctional, reduced, or absent levels of the essential coagulation cofactor, FVIII, with a prevalence of 1/5000 live male births.[41] HA is a monogenic disorder resulting from pathogenic variants that occur in the F8 gene that encodes the FVIII protein. The F8 gene is 187 kb in size and is located on the long arm of the X chromosome at the most distal band (Xq28).[42] F8 is comprises 26 exons ranging in size from 69 bp (exon 26) to 3.1 kb (exon 14) that code for a 9-kb mRNA transcript. Missense mutations are most frequent across all disease severities, with nonsense and splice site variants more frequently associated with severe HA. The remaining unique pathogenic variants associated with HA include deletions (23%), duplications (4.8%), insertions (1.6%), and indels (1.3%).[43] The most common gene defects in severe HA are the intron 1 and intron 22 inversions, which occur in 0% to 5% and 40% to 49% of patients, respectively.[44]

HB is caused by a quantitative or qualitative defect of the coagulation zymogen FIX with a prevalence of 1/30,000 live male births.[41,45] Approximately 50% of HB cases are sporadic, without a known family history.[46] HB is associated exclusively with pathogenic variants located in the F9 gene, which encodes the FIX protein. F9 is located on the long arm of the X chromosome (Xq27), comprises 8 exons, and encodes an mRNA 2.8 kb in length.[47] Most (>70%) of the reported mutations are point mutations; 16% are deletions. The rest are insertions, duplications, and combinations of deletions and insertions.[48,49] A few large rearrangements have also been described.[50] Large deletions, nonsense mutations, and frameshift mutations, resulting from insertions and small deletions, are frequently associated with severe phenotype, whereas missense mutations are associated with severe, moderate, or mild HB.[51]

REFERENCES

1. Khan S, Dickerman JD. Hereditary thrombophilia. Thromb J 2006;4:15.
2. Garcia D, Middeldorp S, Sharathkumar AA. Thrombosis and thrombophilia. Am Soc Hematol Self-Assess Program 2016;2016:185–218.
3. Hollenhorst MA, Battinelli EM. Thrombosis, hypercoagulable states, and anticoagulants. Prim Care 2016;43(4):619–35.
4. De Stefano V, Rossi E, Paciaroni K, et al. Screening for inherited thrombophilia: indications and therapeutic implications. Haematologica 2002;87(10):1095–108.
5. De Stefano V. Inherited thrombophilia and life-time risk of venous thromboembolism: is the burden reducible? J Thromb Haemost 2004;2(9):1522–5.
6. Lane DA, Mannucci PM, Bauer KA, et al. Inherited thrombophilia: part 1. Thromb Haemost 1996;76(5):651–62.
7. Murin S, Marelich GP, Arroliga AC, et al. Hereditary thrombophilia and venous thromboembolism. Am J Respir Crit Care Med 1998;158(5 Pt 1):1369–73.
8. De Stefano V, Finazzi G, Mannucci PM. Inherited thrombophilia: pathogenesis, clinical syndromes, and management. Blood 1996;87(9):3531–44.
9. Miyakis S, Lockshin MD, Atsumi T, et al. International consensus statement on an update of the classification criteria for definite antiphospholipid syndrome (APS). J Thromb Haemost 2006;4(2):295–306.
10. Koike T. Antiphospholipid syndrome: 30 years and our contribution. Int J Rheum Dis 2015;18(2):233–41.
11. Gushiken FC, Arnett FC, Ahn C, et al. Polymorphism of beta2-glycoprotein I at codons 306 and 316 in patients with systemic lupus erythematosus and antiphospholipid syndrome. Arthritis Rheum 1999;42(6):1189–93.
12. Horita T, Atsumi T, Yoshida N, et al. STAT4 single nucleotide polymorphism, rs7574865 G/T, as a risk for antiphospholipid syndrome. Ann Rheum Dis 2009;68(8):1366–7.
13. Otomo K, Atsumi T, Amengual O, et al. Efficacy of the antiphospholipid score for the diagnosis of antiphospholipid syndrome and its predictive value for thrombotic events. Arthritis Rheum 2012;64(2):504–12.

14. de Laat B, Derksen RHWM, Urbanus RT, et al. IgG antibodies that recognize epitope Gly40-Arg43 in domain I of beta 2-glycoprotein I cause LAC, and their presence correlates strongly with thrombosis. Blood 2005;105(4):1540–5.

15. Galli M, Borrelli G, Jacobsen EM, et al. Clinical significance of different antiphospholipid antibodies in the WAPS (warfarin in the antiphospholipid syndrome) study. Blood 2007;110(4):1178–83.

16. Pengo V, Ruffatti A, Legnani C, et al. Clinical course of high-risk patients diagnosed with antiphospholipid syndrome. J Thromb Haemost 2010;8(2):237–42.

17. Flood VH. New insights into genotype and phenotype of VWD. Hematology Am Soc Hematol Educ Program 2014;2014(1):531–5.

18. Johnsen JM, Auer PL, Morrison AC, et al. Common and rare von Willebrand factor (VWF) coding variants, VWF levels, and factor VIII levels in African Americans: the NHLBI exome sequencing project. Blood 2013;122(4):590–7.

19. Flood VH, Gill JC, Morateck PA, et al. Common VWF exon 28 polymorphisms in African Americans affecting the VWF activity assay by ristocetin cofactor. Blood 2010;116(2):280–6.

20. Mancuso DJ, Tuley EA, Westfield LA, et al. Structure of the gene for human von Willebrand factor. J Biol Chem 1989;264(33):19514–27.

21. Mancuso DJ, Tuley EA, Westfield LA, et al. Human von Willebrand factor gene and pseudogene: structural analysis and differentiation by polymerase chain reaction. Biochemistry (Mosc) 1991;30(1):253–69.

22. Wang QY, Song J, Gibbs RA, et al. Characterizing polymorphisms and allelic diversity of von Willebrand factor gene in the 1000 genomes. J Thromb Haemost 2013;11(2):261–9.

23. Bellissimo DB, Christopherson PA, Flood VH, et al. VWF mutations and new sequence variations identified in healthy controls are more frequent in the African-American population. Blood 2012;119(9):2135–40.

24. Sadler JE, Budde U, Eikenboom JCJ, et al. Update on the pathophysiology and classification of von Willebrand disease: a report of the subcommittee on von Willebrand factor. J Thromb Haemost 2006;4(10):2103–14.

25. Leebeek FWG, Eikenboom JCJ. Von Willebrand's disease. N Engl J Med 2016;375(21):2067–80.

26. Lillicrap D. von Willebrand disease: advances in pathogenetic understanding, diagnosis, and therapy. Blood 2013;122(23):3735–40.

27. Ioannidis JP, Ntzani EE, Trikalinos TA, et al. Replication validity of genetic association studies. Nat Genet 2001;29(3):306–9.

28. Othman M, Chirinian Y, Brown C, et al. Functional characterization of a 13-bp deletion (c.-1522_-1510del13) in the promoter of the von Willebrand factor gene in type 1 von Willebrand disease. Blood 2010;116(18):3645–52.

29. Woods AI, Sanchez-Luceros A, Kempfer AC, et al. C1272F: a novel type 2A von Willebrand's disease mutation in A1 domain; its clinical significance. Haemophilia 2012;18(1):112–6.

30. Barrett JC, Clayton DG, Concannon P, et al. Genome-wide association study and meta-analysis find that over 40 loci affect risk of type 1 diabetes. Nat Genet 2009;41(6):703–7.

31. Cooper JD, Smyth DJ, Smiles AM, et al. Meta-analysis of genome-wide association study data identifies additional type 1 diabetes risk loci. Nat Genet 2008;40(12):1399–401.

32. Victor M, Rugeri L, Nougier C, et al. Contribution of genetical analysis for diagnosis of von Willebrand's disease type 2B. Haemophilia 2009;15(2):610–2.

33. Tosetto A, Rodeghiero F, Castaman G, et al. A quantitative analysis of bleeding symptoms in type 1 von Willebrand disease: results from a multicenter European study (MCMDM-1 VWD). J Thromb Haemost 2006;4(4):766–73.

34. Biss TT, Blanchette VS, Clark DS, et al. Quantitation of bleeding symptoms in children with von Willebrand disease: use of a standardized pediatric bleeding questionnaire. J Thromb Haemost 2010;8(5):950–6.

35. Veyradier A, Boisseau P, Fressinaud E, et al. A laboratory phenotype/genotype correlation of 1167 french patients from 670 families with von Willebrand disease: a new epidemiologic picture. Medicine (Baltimore) 2016;95(11):e3038.

36. Hampshire DJ, Goodeve AC. The international society on thrombosis and haematosis von Willebrand disease database: an update. Semin Thromb Hemost 2011;37(5):470–9.

37. Sutherland MS, Cumming AM, Bowman M, et al. A novel deletion mutation is recurrent in von Willebrand disease types 1 and 3. Blood 2009;114(5):1091–8.

38. Peyvandi F, Jayandharan G, Chandy M, et al. Genetic diagnosis of haemophilia and other inherited bleeding disorders. Haemophilia 2006;12(Suppl 3):82–9.

39. Powell JS. Lasting power of new clotting proteins. Hematology Am Soc Hematol Educ Program 2014;2014(1):355–63.

40. Blanchette VS, Key NS, Ljung LR, et al. Definitions in hemophilia: communication from the SSC of the ISTH. J Thromb Haemost 2014;12(11):1935–9.

41. Soucie JM, Evatt B, Jackson D. Occurrence of hemophilia in the United States. The hemophilia surveillance system project investigators. Am J Hematol 1998;59(4):288–94.

42. Gitschier J, Wood WI, Goralka TM, et al. Characterization of the human factor VIII gene. Nature 1984; 312(5992):326–30.

43. Swystun LL, James PD. Genetic diagnosis in hemophilia and von Willebrand disease. Blood Rev 2017; 31(1):47–56.

44. Leiria LB, Roisenberg I, Salzano FM, et al. Introns 1 and 22 inversions and factor VIII inhibitors in patients with severe haemophilia A in southern Brazil. Haemophilia 2009;15(1): 309–13.

45. Plug I, Mauser-Bunschoten EP, Bröcker-Vriends AHJT, et al. Bleeding in carriers of hemophilia. Blood 2006; 108(1):52–6.

46. Goodeve AC. Hemophilia B: molecular pathogenesis and mutation analysis. J Thromb Haemost 2015;13(7):1184–95.

47. Yoshitake S, Schach BG, Foster DC, et al. Nucleotide sequence of the gene for human factor IX (antihemophilic factor B). Biochemistry (Mosc) 1985; 24(14):3736–50.

48. Rallapalli PM, Kemball-Cook G, Tuddenham EG, et al. An interactive mutation database for human coagulation factor IX provides novel insights into the phenotypes and genetics of hemophilia B. J Thromb Haemost 2013;11(7):1329–40.

49. Li T, Miller CH, Payne AB, et al. The CDC Hemophilia B mutation project mutation list: a new online resource. Mol Genet Genomic Med 2013;1(4):238–45.

50. Bowen DJ. Haemophilia A and haemophilia B: molecular insights. Mol Pathol 2002;55(1):1–18.

51. Li T, Miller CH, Driggers J, et al. Mutation analysis of a cohort of US patients with hemophilia B. Am J Hematol 2014;89(4):375–9.

Section II: Anticoagulants

Anticoagulants
Pharmacokinetics, Mechanisms of Action, and Indications

Tracy A. DeWald, PharmD, MHS[a],
Jeffrey B. Washam, PharmD[a], Richard C. Becker, MD[b],*

KEYWORDS

- Anticoagulation • Pharmacokinetics • Mechanism of action • Indication

KEY POINTS

- Patients presenting for elective as well as urgent neurosurgical procedures are commonly receiving anticoagulant therapy.
- Understanding how each anticoagulant agent exerts its activity and the indications for use is important for clinicians when initiating and managing anticoagulant therapy.
- Knowledge of fundamental pharmacokinetic profiles of anticoagulant drugs is necessary to help minimize bleeding and achieve optimal surgical outcomes.

INTRODUCTION

Patients requiring neurosurgical procedures, including elective and emergent surgery, are often receiving an anticoagulant for a non-neurosurgical indication, such as atrial fibrillation, venous thromboembolism, or a mechanical heart valve. To achieve optimal outcomes and minimize the risk of periprocedural bleeding, members of the neurosurgical team must understand and have a sound working knowledge of (1) anticoagulants currently used in patient care; (2) their pharmacokinetic effects, distribution, and potential for drug-drug interactions; and (3) approved clinical indications.

MECHANISM OF ACTION

Treatment options for anticoagulation have increased substantially over the past 10 years with the development and wide-scale availability of oral direct thrombin inhibitors and oral direct factor Xa inhibitors. The addition of these agents to an armamentarium of existing drugs administered intravenously, subcutaneously, or orally has expanded treatment options for thromboprophylaxis and targeted anticoagulation. Differences between these medication classes are summarized and shown in **Fig. 1**.

UNFRACTIONATED HEPARIN

Unfractionated heparin (UFH) is a desirable choice for anticoagulation when a rapid anticoagulant effect is needed due to its rapid onset of action when administered intravenously. UFH is a mixture of sulfated glycosaminoglycans of variable lengths and molecular weights. The anticoagulant effects and pharmacologic properties vary with the size of the molecules.[1,2] UFH exerts its anticoagulant effects in 3 distinct ways. The major anticoagulant effect is the result of its high affinity for antithrombin (AT) and the conformational change in

Disclosure Statement: T.A. DeWald and J.B. Washam report nothing to disclose. R.C. Becker serves as a scientific consultant for Ionis Pharmaceuticals, Bayer and Akcea Therapeutics.

[a] Department of Medicine, Duke Heart Center, DUMC Box 3943, Durham, NC 27710, USA; [b] Department of Medicine, University of Cincinnati Heart, Lung and Vascular Institute, University of Cincinnati College of Medicine, 231 Albert Sabin Way, ML 542, Cincinnati, OH 45267, USA
* Corresponding author.
E-mail address: richard.becker@uc.edu

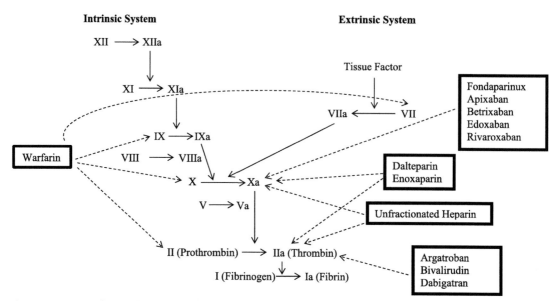

Intrinsic System   **Extrinsic System**

Fig. 1. Overview of coagulation cascade and primary site(s) of action for anticoagulant drugs.

antithrombin (AT) that results from their interaction of heparin and AT. This change accelerates the ability to inactivate the coagulation enzymes thrombin, factor IXa, factor Xa, factor XIa, and factor XIIa. Thrombin and factor Xa are most sensitive to inhibition by the heparin/AT complex; thrombin is approximately 10-fold more sensitive to the inhibiting effects than factor Xa.[1–3] Inhibition of thrombin by UFH requires binding to AT by means of a unique pentasaccharide segment of the heparin molecule and also simultaneous binding of heparin to thrombin by 13 additional saccharide units. Approximately one-third of UFH molecules contain the high-affinity pentasaccharide required for anticoagulant activity.[1,2] The second way in which UFH exerts an anticoagulant effect is through its activity as a catalyst to the inactivation of thrombin by heparin cofactor II. This anticoagulant effect is specific for thrombin and requires much higher doses of UFH than those required to catalyze AT activity.[2] The third anticoagulant effect of UFH is modulation of factor Xa generation, by heparin binding to factor IXa. This effect is not considered clinically significant because it requires dosing of heparin well above those needed for therapeutic efficacy and maintained safety.[1] UFH strongly inhibits thrombin in plasma; the heparin-AT complex is unable to inhibit thrombin bound to fibrin.[1,2]

LOW-MOLECULAR-WEIGHT HEPARINS

Low-molecular-weight heparins (LMWHs) are derived from UFH by means of chemical depolymerization.[1–3] The overall process creates fragments that are approximately one-third the molecular weight of UFH and are also heterogeneous in size.[3] The chemical modification changes several properties of LMWHs. Similar to UFH, LMWHs have a major role in catalyzing AT-mediated inhibition of coagulation factors. However, 50% to 75% of LMWH chains are too short and they experience a progressive loss of ability to catalyze thrombin inhibition.[3,4] These chains, however, are capable of promoting factor Xa inhibition, ultimately leaving LMWHs as more selective inhibitors of factor Xa than UFH.[3] Other distinguishing features of LMWHs from UFH include reduced protein binding that improves their pharmacokinetic properties and results in a more predictable anticoagulant response and reduced interaction with platelets, which results in a reduced formation of heparin-induced thrombocytopenia (HIT) antibodies and incidence of HIT.[3–6]

DIRECT THROMBIN INHIBITORS

Direct thrombin inhibitors interact directly with thrombin; they do not require AT or heparin cofactor II to achieve an anticoagulant effect. They specifically and reversibly inhibit free and clot-bound thrombin by binding to the active site of thrombin.[7–9] Argatroban is classified as a univalent direct thrombin inhibitor, binding only to the catalytic (active) site of thrombin as a competitive inhibitor of thrombin. Bivalirudin is a bivalent thrombin inhibitor, binding to both the catalytic (active) site and the substrate recognition (exosite 1) site of thrombin molecule.[10] Inhibition of thrombin attenuates formation of fibrin, reduces thrombin generation, and may limit platelet activation and aggregation.[11–13] Dabigatran is the only oral direct thrombin inhibitor currently approved by the Food and Drug Administration (FDA) and marketed in the United States.

FACTOR XA INHIBITORS

Fondaparinux was the first of a class of selective inhibitors of factor Xa. It is a chemically synthesized sulfated pentasaccharide that specifically targets AT.[14] After binding to AT, a permanent conformational change occurs in the molecule that causes an increased affinity for factor Xa.[14-16] Fondaparinux does not inhibit thrombin directly, but inactivation of factor Xa by AT provides strong inhibition of thrombin generation.[17,18] Several new direct oral factor Xa inhibitors have been developed and approved by the FDA in the last 10 years. These medications selectively inhibit free and clot-bound factor Xa. They bind directly to the active site of factor Xa, located at the site of convergence of the intrinsic and extrinsic pathways of coagulation, inhibiting free and prothrombinase-bound factor Xa. Binding at this specific site inhibits generation of thrombin, thrombin-mediated activation of coagulation, and thrombin-mediated platelet aggregation.[7,19-22]

WARFARIN

Warfarin exerts its anticoagulant activity through inhibition of the synthesis of vitamin K–dependent coagulation factors II, VII, IX, and X. It also inhibits anticoagulant proteins C and S. Carboxylation of the N-terminal region of the coagulation proteins in the liver is required for their biological activity. Reduced vitamin K is required as a cofactor for their carboxylation.[23] Warfarin interferes with clotting factor synthesis by inhibition of the C1 subunit of vitamin K epoxide reductase enzyme complex, reducing the regeneration of vitamin K_1 epoxide.[23] Recycling of vitamin K is necessary to maintain sufficient intracellular concentrations of vitamin K to serve as a cofactor in the carboxylation. Warfarin (and other coumarin derivatives) inhibit the reductase enzymes responsible for vitamin K recycling, indirectly slowing the rate of synthesis of clotting factors.[24] Therapeutic doses of warfarin reduce the total amount of active vitamin K–dependent clotting factors produced by the liver by 30% to 50%. Warfarin has no direct effect on previously circulating clotting factors or previously formed thrombi.[23-25]

INDICATIONS

Patients receiving anticoagulant medications are commonly encountered in both hospital and ambulatory settings. Having a thorough understanding of the indications for use and the anticoagulant dose and/or intensity recommended is important in situations requiring emergent invasive procedures or life-threatening bleeding events. In the hospital setting, common clinical indications for anticoagulants include prophylaxis of venous thromboembolism in acutely ill medical patients; prophylaxis of venous thromboembolism after surgical procedures, such as knee or hip replacement; thrombosis prophylaxis in patients with acute coronary syndrome; the treatment of acute venous and arterial thromboembolism; and periprocedural anticoagulation during coronary or vascular interventions.

In the ambulatory setting, common indications for oral anticoagulant medications include stroke prophylaxis in patients with atrial fibrillation, thrombosis prophylaxis in patients with mechanical heart valves, treatment and secondary prevention of venous thromboembolism, continuation of venous thromboembolism prophylaxis in patients undergoing knee or hip replacement surgery, and thromboembolism prophylaxis in specific patient populations including those with a known heritable or acquired thrombophilia.

The current FDA-labeled indication(s) for oral anticoagulants and parenteral anticoagulants are shown in **Tables 1** and **2**, respectively.

PHARMACOKINETICS AND DRUG DISPOSITION

The pharmacokinetic characteristics of anticoagulant drugs are presented in **Tables 3** and **4**. Their optimal use incorporates a balance of desired and undesirable medication effects. The magnitudes of both the desired response and toxicity are functions of drug concentration at the site or sites of action.[13] A thorough understanding of medication-specific pharmacokinetic features and potential interactions is essential for optimal prescribing and patient outcome. Medication-specific differences in anticoagulant absorption, distribution, metabolism, and elimination as well disease-specific or condition-specific variations in these fundamental processes govern safe and effect use in clinical practice. Specifically, differences in bioavailability, distribution (including protein binding), metabolism (including cytochrome P450 [CYP450]), and route of elimination may significantly influence drug response.[13] Membrane transporters have become recognized determinants of the pharmacokinetic disposition of many drugs.[26,27] A growing number of membrane transporters have been characterized, with a clinically translatable focus on their expression in the epithelial tissue of intestine, liver, kidney, and

Table 1
Labeled indications for oral anticoagulants

Anticoagulant	Labeled Indication(s)
Warfarin[23]	• Prophylaxis and treatment of venous thrombosis and PE • Prophylaxis and treatment of embolic complications associated with atrial fibrillation or cardiac valve replacement • Reduces the risk of death, recurrent myocardial infarction, and stroke or systemic embolism after myocardial infarction
Apixaban[20]	• Reduces the risk of stroke and systemic embolism in patients with NVAF • Treatment of DVT and PE and for the reduction in the risk of recurrent DVT and PE after initial therapy • DVT prophylaxis in patients who have undergone hip or knee replacement surgery
Betrixaban[19]	• Prophylaxis of VTE in adult patients hospitalized for an acute medical illness who are at risk for thromboembolic complications due to restricted mobility and other risk factors for VTE
Dabigatran[33]	• Reduces the risk of stroke or systemic embolism in patients with NVAF • Treatment of DVT and PE in patients who have been treated with a parenteral anticoagulant for 5–10 d • Reduces the risk of recurrent DVT and PE in patients who have been previously treated • Prophylaxis of DVT and PE in patients who have undergone hip replacement surgery
Edoxaban[21]	• Reduces the risk of stroke and systemic embolism in patients with NVAF • Treatment of DVT and PE after 5–10 d of initial therapy with a parenteral anticoagulant
Rivaroxaban[22]	• Reduces the risk of stroke and systemic embolism in patients with NVAF • Treatment of DVT and PE • Reduces the risk of recurrent DVT and/or PE in patients at continued risk for recurrent DVT and/or PE after completion of initial treatment (at least 6 mo) • Prophylaxis of DVT in patients undergoing hip or knee replacement surgery

Abbreviations: NVAF, nonvalavular atrial fibrillation; VTE, venous thromboembolism.

blood-brain barrier and how they modulate bioavailability and anticoagulant activity.[13,27] The full impact of the growing number of transporters (both efflux and uptake) is unknown at present; however, the role of efflux transporters, specifically permeability glycoprotein (P-gp), is routinely evaluated and documented for many medications in preclinical studies.[27] All oral anticoagulants presented in this review demonstrate that P-gp interactions to some extent have an impact on drug disposition, notably by interaction with other P-gp modulators. Drug substrates for both CYP450 3A4 isoenzyme and P-gp are more likely involved in major drug interactions than drugs that are substrates for only 1 system.[28] Pertinent drug interactions related to P-gp and CYP are summarized in **Table 5**.

The bioavailability of the oral anticoagulants varies widely. For some drugs, the bioavailability changes with coadministration of food. For example, the bioavailability of rivaroxaban (20-mg dose) is 66%.[22] Coadministration of rivaroxaban with food increases the bioavailability of a 20-mg dose, as measured by mean area under the concentration curve (AUC) by 39% and maximum concentration (C_{max}) by 76%.[22] Accordingly, the 15-mg and 20-mg dosage strengths of rivaroxaban should be taken with food (typically the largest meal of the day) and current recommendations suggest administration with the evening meal.[22] The bioavailability of the 10-mg dosage strength is 80% to 100% and does not require food to achieve sufficient concentrations for effective anticoagulation. As such, use of 10-mg rivaroxaban daily for reduction of risk of recurrent deep vein thrombosis (DV)T and/or pulmonary embolism (PE) in patients with continued risk, or for prophylaxis of DVT after hip or knee replacement, may be taken with or without food.[22] Conversely, coadministration of food reduces the bioavailability of betrixaban. The oral bioavailability of betrixaban is 34%, however, consuming a high-fat meal prior to betrixaban administration results in a reduction in both the AUC and C_{max} by 50%, and a reduction in AUC and C_{max} of 70% and 61%, respectively, for a low-fat meal.[19,29] At this time, labeled administration recommendations

Table 2
Labeled indications for parenteral anticoagulants

Anticoagulant	Labeled Indication(s)
UFH[34]	• Prophylaxis and treatment of venous thrombosis and its extension • Prophylaxis and treatment of PE • Prophylaxis and treatment of peripheral arterial embolism • Treatment of acute and chronic consumptive coagulopathies • Atrial fibrillation with embolization • Prevention of clotting in arterial and cardiac surgery • May be used as an anticoagulant in blood transfusions, extracorporeal circulation, and dialysis procedures • Prevention of postoperative DVT and PE in patients undergoing major abdominal surgery who are at risk of developing thromboembolic disease
Enoxaparin[35]	• Prophylaxis of DVT in acutely ill medical patients with severely restricted mobility, abdominal surgery, hip replacement surgery, or knee replacement surgery • Treatment of acute DVT with or without PE • Prophylaxis of ischemic complications in the setting of unstable angina or NSTEMI • Treatment of acute STEMI managed medically or with percutaneous coronary intervention PCI
Dalteparin[36]	• Prophylaxis of ischemic complications of unstable angina or NSTEMI • Prophylaxis of DVT in acutely ill medical patients with severely restricted mobility, abdominal surgery, or hip replacement surgery • Extended treatment of symptomatic venous thromboembolism to reduce recurrence in patients with cancer
Fondaparinux[14]	• Treatment of DVT or PE (in conjunction with warfarin) • Prophylaxis of DVT or PE after orthopedic surgery, including hip replacement, hip fracture, or knee replacement surgery • Prophylaxis of DVT or PE after abdominal surgery in patients who are at risk for thromboembolic complications
Argatroban[8]	• Prophylaxis or treatment of thrombosis in adult patients with HIT • Use as an anticoagulant during PCI in adult patients with or at risk for HIT
Bivalirudin[9]	• Use as an anticoagulant in patients with unstable angina undergoing PTCA • Use as an anticoagulant in patients undergoing PCI with provision use of glycoprotein IIb/IIIa inhibitor • Use as an anticoagulant in patients with or at risk of HIT or HITTS undergoing PCI

Abbreviations: HITTS, HIT and thrombosis syndrome; NSTEMI, non–ST-segment elevation myocardial infarction; PCI, percutaneous coronary intervention; PTCA, percutaneous transluminal coronary angioplasty; STEMI, ST-segment elevation myocardial infarction.

are that betrixaban be taken at the same time each day with food.[19]

The volume of distribution (Vd) varies considerably across the oral anticoagulants. This parameter is a function of drug lipophilicity/tissue affinity, plasma and tissue protein binding affinity, and the presence of active drug transporters on barrier tissues (kidney and liver).[13,30] The differences in Vd explain the extent of tissue distribution of different anticoagulants; however, insufficient information is available at this time to estimate the clinical impact of this difference with respect to patient outcomes.

Finally, drug elimination represents a clinically important variable for consideration when initiating and monitoring anticoagulant therapy. Drug elimination is the process of irreversible removal of drug from the body by all routes of elimination, including biotransformation (metabolism) and drug excretion.[13,30] Enzymes involved in biotransformation are located primarily in the liver where common routes of metabolism include oxidation, reduction, hydrolysis, and conjugation.[13,30]

The CYP450 system is a family of enzymes responsible for most drug metabolism oxidation reactions. Many isoenzymes within this family exist and their role in the metabolism of medications is well established. Although hepatic disease or impairment may result in loss of function that reduces metabolism or elimination of drugs, it is difficult to know when these changes are clinically important and recommendations regarding modification of dosing in the

Table 3
Pharmacokinetic characteristics of oral anticoagulants

	Dabigatran[7,13,33]	Rivaroxaban[7,13,22]	Apixaban[7,13,20]	Edoxaban[7,13,21,37]	Betrixaban[7,19,29,38,39]	Warfarin[23,25,40]
Target	FIIa	FXa	FXa	FXa	FXa	Vitamin K–dependent factors II, VII, IX, and X
Bioavailability	6.5% (absolute)	66% (20-mg dose) increases with food	50% (absolute)	60% (absolute)	34%	80%–100%
Vd	50–70 L	50L	21 L	>107 L (Vd$_{ss}$)	32 L/kg	8–10 L
Protein binding	35%	>90%	87%	40–59	60%	95%–97%
Time to C$_{max}$ (hours)	1–2	2–4	1–4	1–2	3–4	1–2
Half-life (hours)	12–17	5–9	8–15	10–14	19–27	7 d, effective half-life 20–60 h
Hepatic metabolism/ biotransformation	Up to 20% glucuronidation (phase II)	66% undergoes metabolic degradation	30%–35% O-demethylation and hydroxylation major sites (phase I)	Minimal; primarily through conjugation, oxidation by CYP 3A4 and hydrolysis (phase I)	Major biotransformation pathway; via hydrolysis	Major; extensive

Renal excretion Biliary excretion	80% unchanged ~20%	66% (33% direct excretion as unchanged, 33% excreted after metabolic degradation) 28% feces (7% unchanged)	25%–30% 30%–35%	40%–50% 50%	11% Biliary secretion primary route of excretion (via hepatic P-gp) as unchanged drug; 85% recovered in feces.	>90% inactive metabolites
CYP metabolism	No (conjugation)	30%	15%	Yes (% NR)	Minimal <1% (hydrolysis)	Yes
CYP isoenzymes	No	Yes (CYP3A4/5, CYP2J2) Major	Yes CYP3A4/5 Minor (minimal role of CYP1A2, 2C8, 2C9, 2C19, and 2J2)	Yes CYP3A4	< 1% via CYP 1A1, 1A2, 2B6, 2C9, 2C19, 2D6, and 3A4.	Yes 2C9, 2C19, 2C8, 2C18, 1A2, and 3A4 (genetic polymorphism of 2C9 results in variability in response)
Drug transporters	Substrate P-gp (dabigatran etexilate)	Substrate P-gp Substrate ABCG2 (BCRP)	Substrate P-gp Substrate ABCG2 (BCRP)	Substrate P-gp Substrate ABCB1 (MDR1)	Substrate P-gp NR	Substrate and inhibitor of hepatic P-gp ABCB1 (MDR1)

Abbreviations: ABCB1 (MDR1), ATP-binding cassette subfamily B member 1 (multidrug resistance protein 1); ABCG2 (BCRP), ATP-binding cassette subfamily G member 2 (breast cancer resistance protein); FIIa, factor IIa; FXa, factor Xa; NR, not reported Vd_{ss}, Vd at steady state.

Table 4
Pharmacokinetic characteristics of parenteral anticoagulants

	Unfractionated heparin[1,2,34]	Enoxaparin[1,35]	Dalteparin[1,36]	Fondaparinux[14]	Bivalirudin[41,42]	Argatroban[8]
Target	AT	AT	AT	AT	Thrombin	Thrombin
Bioavailability	unpredictable	90%–92% (post-SQ)	87% (SQ)	100% (SQ)	40%–80%	100% IV
Vd	40–70 mL/min (same as blood volume)	4.3 L	3–4 L	7–11 L	0.24 L/Kg	0.174 L/kg
Protein binding	>90%	<UFH	<UFH	≥ 94% specifically to ATIII	No plasma proteins; just thrombin	55% 20% albumin 35% α-acid glycoprotein
Time to peak activity (hours)	Rapid after bolus, 4–6 h after infusion	3–5 h (SQ) (pk anti-Xa activity)	2–4 h (SQ) (pk anti-Xa activity)	2–3 h (SQ) (pk steady-state concentration)	2 min after bolus; 4 min after 15 min infusion (pk plasma concentrations)	3–4 h after infusion (pk plasma concentrations)
Half-life (hours)	1.0–1.5 (infusion)	5.0 (prolonged in severe RI, and with repeated dosing)	3–5 (prolonged in RI)	17 (young) 21 (elderly)	0.5 (prolonged in moderate–severe RI)	0.5–1.0
Elimination	Primarily by reticuloendothelial system. Small fraction excreted in urine.	80% Renal	Renal	Renal	Renal and proteolytic cleavage	Hepatic hydroxylation; 16% renal excretion as unchanged drug 14% biliary excretion as unchanged drug
CYP metabolism	No	No	No	No	No	Yes
CYP isoenzymes	No	No	No	No	No	CYP 3A4/5; not believed to contribute significantly

Abbreviations: anti-Xa, anti-factor Xa; CI, continuous infusion; pk, peak; RI, renal insufficiency; SQ, subcutaneous.

Table 5
Drug-drug interactions for oral anticoagulant agents

Medication	Interactions[a]	Management
Apixaban[20]	• Strong dual CYP3A4 and P-gp inducers (eg, rifampin, carbamazepine, phenytoin, and St. John's wort) • Strong dual CYP3A4 and P-gp inhibitors (eg, ketoconazole, itraconazole, ritonavir, and clarithromycin)	• Avoid concomitant use • In patients taking 5 mg twice daily of apixaban, reduce dose to 2.5 mg twice daily. In patients taking 2.5 mg twice daily, avoid, concomitant use.
Betrixaban[19]	• P-gp inhibitors (eg, amiodarone, azithromycin, verapamil, ketoconazole, and clarithromycin)	• Reduce dose of betrixaban in patients receiving a P-gp inhibitor. Avoid concomitant use of betrixaban and P-gp inhibitor in patients with severe renal dysfunction (CrCL 15–29 mL/min).
Dabigatran[33]	• P-gp inducers (eg, rifampin) • P-gp inhibitors (eg, ketoconazole and dronedarone)	• Avoid concomitant use • For indication of stroke prophylaxis in AF: In patients with moderate renal impairment (CrCl 30–50 mL/min), reduce dabigatran dose to 75 mg twice daily. Avoid in patients with severe renal impairment (CrCl 15–30 mL/min). • For indication of treatment and reduction in the risk of recurrence of DVT and PE; avoid concomitant use of dabigatran and P-gp inhibitors in patients with CrCl <50 mL/min. • For indication of prophylaxis of DVT and PE after hip replacement surgery: in patients with CrCl >50 mL/min taking P-gp inhibitors, such as dronedarone or ketoconazole, consider separating the administration timing of dabigatran and the P-gp inhibitor by several hours. Avoid concomitant use of dabigatran and P-gp inhibitors in patients with CrCl <50 mL/min.

(continued on next page)

Table 5
(continued)

Medication	Interactions[a]	Management
Edoxaban[21]	• P-gp inducers (eg, rifampin)	• Avoid concomitant use.
Rivaroxaban[22]	• Strong dual CYP3A4 and P-gp inducers (eg, carbamazepine, phenytoin, rifampin, and St. John's wort) • Strong dual CYP3A4 and P-gp inhibitors (eg, ketoconazole, ritonavir) • Moderate dual CYP3A4 and P-gp inhibitors (eg, erythromycin) in patients with renal impairment (CrCl 15 mL/min to <80 mL/min)	• Avoid concomitant use. • Avoid concomitant administration. • Rivaroxaban should not be used in patients with CrCl 15 mL/min to <80 mL/min concomitantly with combined P-gp and moderate CYP3A4 inhibitors unless the potential benefit justifies the potential risk.
Warfarin[43]	• Medications highly probable of warfarin potentiation (eg, ciprofloxacin, cotrimoxazole, erythromycin, fluconazole, isoniazid, metronidazole, miconazole, voriconazole, amiodarone, clofibrate, diltiazem, fenofibrate, propafenone, propranolol, sulfinpyrazone, phenylbutazone, piroxicam, citalopram, entacapone, sertraline, cimetidine, omeprazole, anabolic steroids, zileuton) • Medications highly probable of warfarin inhibition (eg, griseofulvin, nafcillin, ribavirin, rifampin, cholestyramine, mesalamine, barbiturates, carbamazepine, and mercaptopurine)	• Avoid if possible. If concomitant therapy must be used, increase the frequency of monitoring and adjust the warfarin dose based on the INR results. • Avoid if possible. If concomitant therapy must be used, increase the frequency of monitoring and adjust the warfarin dose based on the INR results.

Abbreviations: AF, atrial fibrillation; CrCl, creatinine clearance; INR, international normalized ratio.

[a] Interactions listed are those offered as examples and are not intended to be a comprehensive listing of all possible interacting medications; for complete listing of interactions, please refer to approved package labeling.

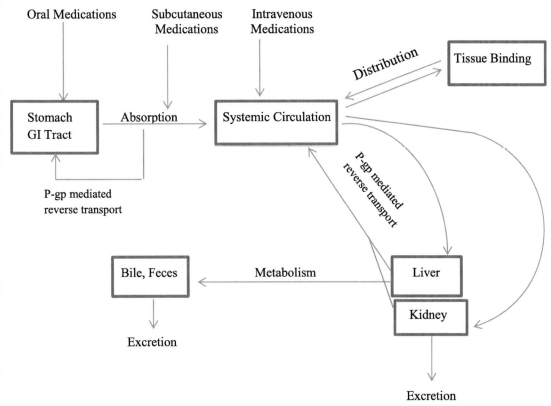

Fig. 2. Overview of drug pharmacokinetic process. Note the complete role of transporters in absorption, disposition, excretion, and drug-drug interactions because they might contribute to clinical consequences is not fully known.

setting of hepatic impairment are nonspecific and difficult to apply.[31] Understanding the primary route of metabolism and elimination may assist in the selection of preferred anticoagulant therapy.

In addition to metabolism and biotransformation, drugs are eliminated by excretion into bile or into urine.[13] The processes by which a drug is excreted by the kidneys may include any combination of glomerular filtration, active tubular secretion, or tubular reabsorption.[13,30] In the presence of renal disease, both glomerular filtration and renal tubular secretion can decrease, impairing the renal clearance of drugs and their metabolites.[13,32] The degree to which impairment in these processes prolongs the presence or half-life of a drug, potentially extending the pharmacodynamics effect, is dependent on the proportion of drug excreted by the renal route of elimination and the extent of renal impairment.[13,32] Knowledge of anticoagulant-specific reliance on the renal route of elimination can guide preferred treatment choices and tailor individualized monitoring plans. A brief overview of the pharmacokinetic process is displayed in **Fig. 2**.

SUMMARY

Anticoagulants are widely used for a variety of diseases, disorders, and conditions. The availability of oral anticoagulant treatment options has expanded greatly in the past 10 years, mostly with the development of direct thrombin inhibition and factor Xa inhibition. There are important differences in indications, pharmacokinetic profiles, and interaction potentials among anticoagulants. Tailored therapy for individual patient needs and procedures is essential for optimizing anticoagulation outcomes and minimizing procedural complications.

REFERENCES

1. Hirsh J, Bauer KA, Donati MB, et al. Parenteral anticoagulants: American College of Chest Physicians evidence-based clinical practice guidelines (8th Edition). Chest 2008;133(6 Suppl):141S–59S.
2. Hirsh J, Raschke R, Warkentin TE, et al. Heparin: mechanism of action, pharmacokinetics, dosing considerations, monitoring, efficacy, and safety. Chest 1995;108(4 Suppl):258S–75S.

3. Garcia DA, Baglin TP, Weitz JI, et al. Parenteral anticoagulants: antithrombotic therapy and prevention of thrombosis, 9th ed: American College of Chest Physicians evidence-based clinical practice guidelines. Chest 2012;141(2 Suppl):e24S–43S.

4. Weitz JI. Low-molecular-weight heparins. N Engl J Med 1997;337(10):688–98.

5. Warkentin TE, Levine MN, Hirsh J, et al. Heparin-induced thrombocytopenia in patients treated with low-molecular-weight heparin or unfractionated heparin. N Engl J Med 1995;332(20):1330–5.

6. Cosmi B, Fredenburgh JC, Rischke J, et al. Effect of nonspecific binding to plasma proteins on the antithrombin activities of unfractionated heparin, low-molecular-weight heparin, and dermatan sulfate. Circulation 1997;95(1):118–24.

7. Eriksson BI, Quinlan DJ, Weitz JI. Comparative pharmacodynamics and pharmacokinetics of oral direct thrombin and factor xa inhibitors in development. Clin Pharmacokinet 2009;48(1):1–22.

8. Argatroban. (argatroban) [prescribing information]. Research Triangle Park (NC): GlaxoSmithKline; 2016.

9. Angiomax. (bivalirudin) [prescribing information]. Parsippany (NJ): The Medicines Company; 2016.

10. Kam PC, Kaur N, Thong CL. Direct thrombin inhibitors: pharmacology and clinical relevance. Anaesthesia 2005;60(6):565–74.

11. Mann KG. Thrombin formation. Chest 2003; 124(3 Suppl):4S–10S.

12. Weitz JI. Factor Xa and thrombin as targets for new oral anticoagulants. Thromb Res 2011;127(Suppl 2): S5–12.

13. DeWald TA, Becker RC. The pharmacology of novel oral anticoagulants. J Thromb Thrombolysis 2014; 37(2):217–33.

14. Arixtra. (fondaparinux) [prescribing information]. Rockford (IL): Mylan Institutional, LLC; 2017.

15. Bauer KA, Hawkins DW, Peters PC, et al. Fondaparinux, a synthetic pentasaccharide: the first in a new class of antithrombotic agents - the selective factor Xa inhibitors. Cardiovasc Drug Rev 2002; 20(1):37–52.

16. Cheng JW. Fondaparinux: a new antithrombotic agent. Clin Ther 2002;24(11):1757–69 [discussion: 1719].

17. Walenga JM, Bara L, Petitou M, et al. The inhibition of the generation of thrombin and the antithrombotic effect of a pentasaccharide with sole anti-factor Xa activity. Thromb Res 1988;51(1):23–33.

18. Lormeau JC, Herault JP. The effect of the synthetic pentasaccharide SR 90107/ORG 31540 on thrombin generation ex vivo is uniquely due to ATIII-mediated neutralization of factor Xa. Thromb Haemost 1995; 74(6):1474–7.

19. Bevyxxa. (betrixaban) [prescribing information]. San Francisco (CA): Portola Pharmaceuticals, Inc; 2017.

20. Eliquis. (apixaban) [prescribing information]. Princeton (NJ): Bristol-Myers Squibb Company; 2018.

21. Savaysa. (edoxaban) [prescribing information]. Basking Ridge (NJ): Daiichi Sankyo, Inc; 2017.

22. Xarelto. (rivaroxaban) [prescribing information]. Titusville (NJ): Janssen Pharmaceuticals, Inc; 2017.

23. Coumadin. (warfarin) [prescribing information]. Princeton (NJ): Bristol-Myers Squibb Company; 2017.

24. Stirling Y. Warfarin-induced changes in procoagulant and anticoagulant proteins. Blood Coagul Fibrinolysis 1995;6(5):361–73.

25. Hirsh J. Oral anticoagulant drugs. N Engl J Med 1991;324(26):1865–75.

26. Zhang DLG, Ding X, Lu C. Preclinical experimental models of drug metabolism and disposition in drug discovery and development. Acta Pharm Sin B 2012;2(6):549–61.

27. International Transporter C, Giacomini KM, Huang SM, et al. Membrane transporters in drug development. Nat Rev Drug Discov 2010;9(3): 215–36.

28. Zhang Y, Benet LZ. The gut as a barrier to drug absorption: combined role of cytochrome P450 and P-glycoprotein. Clin Pharmacokinet 2001; 40(3):159–68.

29. Chan NC, Hirsh J, Ginsberg JS, et al. Betrixaban (PRT054021): pharmacology, dose selection and clinical studies. Future Cardiol 2014;10(1):43–52.

30. Shargel L. Applied biopharmaceutics and pharmacokinetics. 3rd edition. Norwalk (CT): Appleton and Lange; 1993.

31. Verbeeck R. Pharmacokinetics and dosage adjustment in patients with hepatic dysfunction. Eur J Clin Pharmacol 2008;64(12):1147–61.

32. Matzke GR, Aronoff GR, Atkinson AJ Jr, et al. Drug dosing consideration in patients with acute and chronic kidney disease-a clinical update from Kidney Disease: Improving Global Outcomes (KDIGO). Kidney Int 2011;80(11):1122–37.

33. Pradaxa. (dabigatran) [prescribing information]. Ridgefield (CT): Boehringer Ingelheim Pharmaceuticals, Inc; 2017.

34. Heparin. (heparin sodium for injection) [prescribing information]. Lake Forest (IL): Hospira, Inc; 2016.

35. Lovenox. (enoxaparin sodium) [prescribing information]. Bridgewater (NJ): Sanofi-Aventis US LLC; 2017.

36. Fragmin. (dalteparin sodium) [prescribing information]. New York: Pfizer Labs; 2017.

37. Bathala MS, Masumoto H, Oguma T, et al. Pharmacokinetics, biotransformation, and mass balance of edoxaban, a selective, direct factor Xa inhibitor, in humans. Drug Metab Dispos 2012;40(12):2250–5.

38. Leeds JMKA, Yeo KR, Curnutte JT, et al. Physiologically based pharmacokinetic (PBPK) modeling for betrixaban and the impact of p-glycoprotein

inhibition on betrixaban pharmackinetics. Blood 2017;130(Suppl 1):3663.

39. Hutchaleelaha AYC, Song Y, Lorenz T, et al. Metabolism and disposition of betrixaban and its lack of interaction with major cyp enzymes [abstract]. Blood 2012;120(21):2266.

40. Holford NH. Clinical pharmacokinetics and pharmacodynamics of warfarin. Understanding the dose-effect relationship. Clin Pharmacokinet 1986;11(6): 483–504.

41. Fox I, Dawson A, Loynds P, et al. Anticoagulant activity of Hirulog, a direct thrombin inhibitor, in humans. Thromb Haemost 1993;69(2):157–63.

42. Gladwell TD. Bivalirudin: a direct thrombin inhibitor. Clin Ther 2002;24(1):38–58.

43. Ageno W, Gallus AS, Wittkowsky A, et al. Oral anticoagulant therapy: antithrombotic therapy and prevention of thrombosis, 9th ed: American College of Chest Physicians evidence-based clinical practice guidelines. Chest 2012;141(2 Suppl):e44S–88S.

Use of Antiplatelet Agents in the Neurosurgical Patient

Amanda S. Zakeri, MD, Shahid M. Nimjee, MD, PhD*

KEYWORDS

- Antiplatelet • Neurosurgery • Aneurysms • Carotid dissection • Carotid stenosis
- Moyamoya disease • Stroke

KEY POINTS

- Antiplatelet therapy is an important part of treating vascular neurologic conditions including carotid artery disease and dissection, intracranial atherosclerotic disease, and moyamoya disease.
- Technological advances in endovascular neurosurgery to treat intracranial aneurysms have resulted in antiplatelet agents being used uniformly electively and increasingly in the acute setting.
- Ischemic stroke has evolved in part to an interventional disease. Medical management may include dual antiplatelet therapy (DAPT) acutely and certainly monotherapy chronically.

INTRODUCTION

Antiplatelet therapy has long been used in a variety of neurosurgical vascular conditions. This article presents relevant literature on the role of antiplatelet therapy in neurosurgical vascular diseases. There is a significant challenge in broadly recommending one or even multiple agents over others. Current literature supports developing an individualized approach to each patient. It is hoped that this serves as a starting point for readers to better understand which regimens have the best evidence to support their implementation in clinical practice and which areas are still under active investigation.

ANEURYSMS

Coil Embolization and Stent-Assisted Coil Embolization for Intracranial Aneurysms

There are currently no randomized clinical trials (RCTs) or published guidelines to support a specific therapeutic regimen or duration of therapy following endovascular treatment of either ruptured or unruptured aneurysms treated with stent-assisted embolization.[1] Because of the risk of thrombosis associated with stent placement, antiplatelet therapy has played an essential role in preventing complications associated with stent-assisted coiling of intracranial arteries. Aspirin (81 or 325 mg) and clopidogrel (75 mg) are commonly used following stent placement but optimal duration of therapy is unknown.

In the setting of unruptured aneurysms treated electively, a retrospective study by Choi and colleagues[2] found that pretreatment with low-dose prasugrel had better efficacy in comparison with clopidogrel for prevention of thrombotic complications without a significant difference in the rate of hemorrhagic events. Patients in the prasugrel group had significantly lower P2Y12 reaction unit (PRU) values and a higher percentage of platelet inhibition. Another retrospective review found 5% increased risk of ischemic events following discontinuation of clopidogrel after 6 weeks.[3] Despite these findings, RCT are necessary to

Disclosure Statement: The authors have nothing to disclose.
Department of Neurological Surgery, Ohio State University Medical Center, N-1014 Doan Hall, 410 West 10th Avenue, Columbus, OH 43210, USA
* Corresponding author.
E-mail address: shahid.nimjee@osumc.edu

Neurosurg Clin N Am 29 (2018) 517–527
https://doi.org/10.1016/j.nec.2018.06.004
1042-3680/18/© 2018 Elsevier Inc. All rights reserved.

determine whether prasugrel provides true benefit over clopidogrel, and ideal duration of therapy remains to be determined.

Antiplatelet therapy may reduce the risk of thromboembolism when administered before or during stent-assisted endovascular treatment of ruptured intracranial aneurysms. A meta-analysis performed by Ryu and colleagues[4] found a greater risk of thromboembolism in patients with ruptured aneurysms compared with unruptured aneurysms when antiplatelet therapy was not administered until after completion of the procedure. There was no increased risk of thrombosis for patients who received either a preprocedural loading dose of aspirin and clopidogrel or modified therapy with glycoprotein (GP) IIb/IIIa inhibitors after stent deployment. It is worth noting that among patients undergoing percutaneous coronary interventions, the addition of short-term intravenous infusion of GP IIb/IIIa antagonists reduced the risk of early arterial or stent thrombosis in large RCTs.[5] This benefit was evident for at least the first month, but more recent evidence suggests that it may persist for at least 6 months.[6–9] In light of these findings, in addition to the review performed by Dornbos and colleagues, it may be beneficial to incorporate the use of GP IIb/IIIa inhibitors when endovascular intervention is indicated for treatment of intracranial aneurysms.

Pipeline Flow Diversion

In 2011, the pipeline embolization device (PED; ev3, Plymouth, MA) was approved for treatment of intracranial aneurysms. Initially, flow diversion with PED gained favor in treatment of aneurysms with morphology unfavorable to current open neurosurgical and endovascular embolization techniques.[10] Specifically, it initially provided an effective alternative approach for large, giant, and nonsaccular aneurysms.[10,11] Now, the role of PED in neurointerventions has expanded to include small, fusiform, and saccular aneurysms.

Although an effective treatment, flow diversion stent treatment of aneurysms has been associated with a widely variable risk of thromboembolic (0%–14%) and hemorrhagic (0%–11%) complications.[12] Because of the risk of thrombosis, antiplatelet therapy is essential and a wide variety of treatment strategies have been used without clear evidence of an ideal treatment regimen (**Table 1**).[13] The most common post-PED treatment involved aspirin for at least 6 months in addition to clopidogrel for 3 to 12 months (93% of 1180 patients) with longer duration after PED procedures in the posterior circulation (see **Table 1**).[13] Despite use of dual antiplatelet therapy (DAPT) before and following the procedure, there remains a significant risk of thromboembolic complications (TEC) related to variable therapeutic responses to the standard regimen.[14,15]

Routine assessment of preoperative platelet function test (PFT) is not consistently performed at every center, yet multiple studies have shown potential benefit before treatment with PED.[12,14,16–19] Current methods for this purpose included VerifyNow to obtain PRU with or without aspirin reaction units, light transmission aggregometry to assess aspirin and ADP inhibition percentiles, and/or multiplate platelet-aggregation test to measure aggregation units.[13] Although one systematic review did not find a statistically significant difference in TEC related to PFT, there was a trend toward increased risk of TEC in patients who received no form of PFT.[13] Specifically, one study found an increased risk of thrombotic and hemorrhagic complications associated with PRU greater than 240 or less than 60, respectively, and recommended that target PRU values before PED placement should lie between 60 and 240 and ideally between 70 and 150.[14] Given the lack of formal guidelines, we recommend the routine use of PFT before treatment with PED.

The potential need for PFT is in part caused by the risk for insufficient response to clopidogrel,

Table 1
Preprocedural antiplatelet regimen

Percentage of Patients	Number of Patients	Aspirin Dose (mg)	Aspirin Duration (d)	Clopidogrel Dose (mg)	Clopidogrel Duration (d)
61.7	803	300–325	2–14	75	3 to >10
21.7	351	81	5–10	75	5–10
6.3	82	100–150	5	75	5

Percentage of patients reflects percentage of 1300 patients identified in systematic review whose intracranial aneurysms were treated by PED.

Data from Texakalidis P, Bekelis K, Atallah E, et al. Flow diversion with the pipeline embolization device for patients with intracranial aneurysms and antiplatelet therapy: a systematic literature review. Clin Neurol Neurosurg 2017;161:78–87.

because approximately 30% of patients are biochemically resistant.[20] Nonresponse to clopidogrel has been associated with a significantly increased risk of TEC, which was ameliorated when patients were provided with additional antiplatelet medication before procedure.[16] Thus, in the case of allergy, resistance (defined as <30% of platelet P2Y12 receptor inhibition), or nonresponse to clopidogrel or aspirin, other antiplatelet agents may be beneficial to reduce the risk of TEC. Current options of alternative DAPT include P2Y12 inhibitors (prasugrel or ticagrelor) and ADP receptor blocker (ticlopidine). Another strategy to reduce the incidence of TEC is the use of loading doses of the previously mentioned and/or aspirin or clopidogrel shortly before the procedure.[13,16,17] The use of GP IIb/IIIa inhibitors has also been evaluated in the setting of prophylaxis for TEC when patients were unable to receive preoperative DAPT and in acute intraoperative thrombosis and was found to be safe and effective.[9,21] However, further RCT are necessary to determine routine use of these agents for prophylaxis.

CAROTID DISSECTION

Extracranial carotid artery dissection poses a significant risk for ipsilateral stroke at presentation, and a high risk for recurrent stroke following detection, particularly in patients who present with acute ischemic stroke (AIS) or transient ischemic attack (TIA).[22–24] Although only 1% to 2% of ischemic strokes are caused by carotid dissection, it accounts for approximately 10% to 25% of ischemic strokes in young and middle-aged patients.[25] Both anticoagulation and antiplatelet therapy has been used in the setting of acute extracranial carotid artery dissection to prevent TEC.

The Cervical Artery Dissection in Stroke Study (CADISS) was the first RCT performed to directly compare these therapies in patients with symptomatic cervical artery dissection.[22] The authors found that there was no difference in efficacy for preventing stroke or death, nor was there a difference in rates of major bleeding between antiplatelet versus anticoagulant therapy. The choice of antiplatelet therapy was left to the discretion of the local physician and included aspirin, dipyridamole, or clopidogrel alone or in combination. The most commonly used treatments included aspirin alone (28 patients; 22%), clopidogrel alone (42 patients; 33%), aspirin with clopidogrel (35 patients; 28%), and aspirin with dipyridamole (20 patients; 16%) each for 3 months. The authors note that there may have been improved efficacy of stroke prevention had all patients received DAPT; however, considering the rarity of stroke (3 patients; 2%)

the addition of a second antiplatelet therapy may not be worth the potential increased risk of major hemorrhage. In addition, a prospective, nonrandomized study of 298 patients (96 treated with aspirin alone) found that the frequency of ischemic events did not differ significantly in patients treated with anticoagulation versus aspirin alone.[24] Because of the limited number of postdissection strokes in patients receiving either therapy, larger studies are necessary to determine optimal medical therapy and duration of treatment.

The 2018 American Heart Association (AHA) guidelines for AIS suggest that for patients with AIS and extracranial carotid or vertebral arterial dissection, treatment with either antiplatelet or anticoagulant therapy for 3 to 6 months may be reasonable (COR IIB, LOE B-R).[26] The Society for Vascular Surgery recommends initial management with antithrombotic therapy (antiplatelet agents or anticoagulation) (grade 1, LOE C).[27] For patients who experience persistent ischemic neurologic symptoms despite medical therapy intervention with balloon angioplasty and stenting may be considered (grade 2, LOE C)[27] (class IIB, LOE C).[28]

CAROTID ARTERY STENOSIS
Asymptomatic Extracranial Carotid Artery Stenosis

Carotid artery occlusive disease accounts for approximately 20% of ischemic strokes.[29] In one early study, approximately 80% of patients with first stroke were asymptomatic before presentation and had no prior history of stroke or TIA.[30] Although some studies have cited increased risk of vascular events and death[31] in patients with asymptomatic carotid atherosclerotic disease, more recent evidence suggests that patients treated with intensive contemporary medical therapy alone have an annual risk of stroke less than or equal to 1%.[32–34] Nonetheless, there is limited evidence to support the routine use of antiplatelet therapy for primary prevention of stroke.[35–37]

Current guidelines from the AHA for primary prevention of stroke in asymptomatic carotid artery stenosis (ACAS) recommend daily aspirin (class I, LOE C).[38] In addition, the Society for Vascular Surgery recommends antiplatelet therapy to reduce overall cardiovascular morbidity (grade 1, LOE A). The 2011 guidelines for management of patients with extracranial carotid disease also endorse antiplatelet therapy with aspirin, 75 to 325 mg daily, for prevention of myocardial infarction (MI) and other ischemic cardiovascular events (class I, LOE A). The US Preventive Services Task Force recommends daily aspirin for reduction of cardiovascular events in patients with anticipated cardiac morbidity of greater than 3% for men older than 45 years and women older than 55 years. The most common doses of aspirin prescribed for long-term prevention of cardiovascular disease are 81 mg (60%) and 325 mg (35%) per day.[39] There is currently insufficient data to support the long-term use of dosages greater than 75 to 81 mg per day.[39]

For patients allergic to aspirin, clopidogrel monotherapy has been recommended.[40] In patients who have an allergy or contraindication to aspirin therapy, other than active bleeding, either clopidogrel (75 mg daily) or ticlopidine (250 mg twice daily) have been recommended as reasonable alternatives (class IIa, LOE C).[28]

According to one review, there is currently no evidence to support the use of DAPT or antiplatelet therapy other than aspirin for ACAS.[27] The Clopidogrel for High Atherothrombotic Risk and Ischemic Stabilization, Management and Avoidance (CHARISMA) study demonstrated that in asymptomatic patients with greater than or equal to 70% carotid artery stenosis the use of clopidogrel plus aspirin failed to reduce the incidence of MI, stroke, or cardiovascular death and was associated with an increased risk of cardiovascular death and bleeding.[41] DAPT with aspirin and clopidogrel has been recommended for patients with concomitant symptomatic coronary artery disease, recent coronary stenting, and severe peripheral arterial disease.[40] However, this recommendation is controversial because some studies have shown a reduction of vascular events in patients with acute coronary syndromes,[42,43] whereas others have shown no significant benefit for prevention of cardiovascular events among patients at high risk for cardiovascular disease, or those with symptomatic carotid stenosis, prior stroke, or TIA.[41,44]

The Carotid Artery Stenosis with Asymptomatic Narrowing: Operation versus Aspirin (CASANOVA) study was the first randomized trial to assess the efficacy of prophylactic carotid endarterectomy (CEA) in addition to antiplatelet therapy for the prevention of stroke in patients with ACAS of 50% to 90%.[45] The authors did not detect a significant benefit in patients treated prophylactically with CEA and did not recommend CEA for asymptomatic patients with stenosis less than 90%. However, a more recent randomized trial found significant long-term benefit following CEA for ACAS greater than or equal to 50% when the risk of perioperative stroke and death are less than or equal to 3%.[36] Other studies including ACAS and Asymptomatic Carotid Surgery Trial (ACST) can be discussed; however, surgery provides marginal benefit and only in a highly selected subgroup of patients. These studies were also limited by a suboptimal medical treatment arm that was not uniformly defined.[40] In addition, the current AHA guidelines for primary prevention of stroke acknowledge that randomized trials have shown that prophylactic CEA can provide reduced risk of stroke in appropriately selected patients, despite limited absolute risk reduction. However, they note that contemporary medical management has improved since these studies were performed and the benefit of revascularization may be reduced or even negated with current medical therapy.[32,38]

Symptomatic Extracranial Carotid Artery Stenosis

Patients with symptomatic carotid artery stenosis vary greatly from patients with asymptomatic carotid atherosclerosis because of a significantly greater risk of stroke following presentation with either TIA or stroke.[46] Among patients presenting with TIA or minor stroke there is significantly increased risk of ipsilateral stroke within the first 90 days, and especially within the first 30 days.[47] This risk is reduced by up to 80% with prompt initiation of treatment.[47] Antiplatelet therapy plays a vital role in treatment; however, the ideal medication, dose, and duration of therapy varies depending on whether patients are treated with medical therapy alone, CEA, or carotid artery stenting (CAS). For recommendations regarding antiplatelet therapy in the setting of acute stroke and patients with symptomatic carotid stenosis less than 50% or those not undergoing revascularization procedures see the section on stroke later in the article for discussion of medical therapy. To limit redundancy, this section focuses on recommendations regarding the use of antiplatelet therapy in the perioperative and postoperative period following CEA and CAS.

For neurologically symptomatic patients with stenosis less than 50%, optimal medical therapy is indicated and there are no data to support revascularization procedures (grade 1, LOE B).[27] In general, for patients with symptomatic carotid artery stenosis who are candidates for revascularization, CEA is preferred to CAS for reducing the risk of stroke and periprocedural death (grade 1, LOE B).[27] In addition, patients presenting with stroke or TIA should undergo revascularization with CEA within 2 weeks of presentation for prevention of secondary stroke.[48]

Carotid Endarterectomy

Antiplatelet therapy before CEA significantly reduces the risk of thromboembolic stroke in the perioperative setting. The Society for Vascular Surgery recommends aspirin (81–325 mg) (grade 1, LOE A) with the use of clopidogrel decided on a case-by-case basis (grade 2, LOE B).[27] For patients already taking aspirin therapy, discontinuation before surgery is not necessary nor is it recommended because of increased risk of periprocedural MI related to aspirin withdrawal.[27] DAPT is not recommended for patients without medical necessity (eg, prior placement of drug-eluting stents) because of increased risk of major bleeding compared with aspirin or clopidogrel monotherapy.[44,49] There are insufficient data to adequately assess the risk-benefit profile of continued clopidogrel monotherapy in the perioperative period for CEA.[27] Following CEA it is recommended that patients remain on aspirin indefinitely for secondary prevention of stroke.[8,27,48,50–52] Nonetheless, other guidelines have recommended the use of aspirin (75–325 mg daily), clopidogrel (75 mg daily), or the combination of low-dose aspirin in addition to extended-release dipyridamole (25 and 200 mg twice daily) for long-term prevention of ischemic cardiovascular events in patients 30 days out from CEA (class 1, LOE B).[28]

Carotid Artery Stenting

Despite the increasingly frequent use of CAS for treatment of extracranial carotid artery disease, there remains a paucity of evidence to suggest a definitive duration of antiplatelet therapy following intervention. Current recommendations involve the use of DAPT before and for the first month after CAS placement followed by monotherapy with aspirin. The utility of DAPT was supported by the Clopidogrel and Aspirin for Reduction of Emboli in Symptomatic Carotid Stenosis (CARESS) trial, which demonstrated a reduction in microemboli among patients treated with both clopidogrel and aspirin compared with aspirin monotherapy.[53] Although other authors have attempted to directly apply the results of studies assessing DAPT versus antiplatelet monotherapy in TIA or stroke (eg, MATCH, CHARISMA) to patients undergoing CAS, there remains a significant difference between these populations. During revascularization with CAS, patients are predisposed to additional risk of ischemic stroke secondary to distal emboli from plaque rupture and formation of a mural thrombus related to intravascular catheter manipulation and placement of a foreign body within the vessel.[54,55] Thus, the potential benefit from DAPT for CAS may outweigh the increased bleeding risk found in those studies.

INTRACRANIAL ATHEROSCLEROTIC DISEASE/STENOSIS

Atherosclerosis of the major intracranial arteries is an important risk factor for stroke and is also associated with a significant risk of subsequent ischemic stroke.[56–58] Earlier studies found that warfarin was superior to aspirin for the prevention of major vascular events in the treatment of symptomatic ICA.[57] However, Warfarin-Aspirin Symptomatic Intracranial Disease (WASID), an RCT, provided evidence to suggest that aspirin (1300 mg daily) was equally efficacious to warfarin (target international normalized ratio, 2.0–3.0) for treatment of symptomatic intracranial atherosclerotic disease (ICAD). In fact, it was preferred over warfarin in this patient population because of increased risk of adverse events with warfarin, which prompted cessation of enrollment.[59] Moreover, the AHA guidelines recommend the use of antiplatelet agents rather than oral anticoagulation to reduce the risk of stroke and other cardiovascular events in patients with noncardioembolic AIS (COR I, LOE A). For patients with noncardioembolic stroke while taking antiplatelet therapy, the guidelines do not recommend switching to warfarin for secondary stroke prevention (COR III, LOE B-R). This is supported by a post hoc analysis from WASID that found no difference in primary outcomes of patients who were randomized to warfarin despite taking antiplatelet therapy at the time of their qualifying event.[60,61]

The Stenting versus Aggressive Medical Management for Preventing Recurrent Stroke in Intracranial Stenosis (SAMMPRIS) trial investigated the role of stenting versus aggressive medical management of patients with recent TIA or stroke attributed to 70% to 99% stenosis of a major intracranial artery.[62] Antiplatelet therapy in both groups included aspirin, 325 mg daily, plus clopidogrel, 75 mg daily, for 90 days. In addition, patients who were not taking clopidogrel, 75 mg daily, for at least 5 days before percutaneous transluminal angioplasty and stenting were given a loading dose (600 mg) of clopidogrel 6 to 24 hours before the procedure. The study was stopped early because of a significantly increased risk of stroke or death within the first 30 days following intervention and the authors concluded that aggressive medical management was superior to stenting with the wingspan device for secondary prevention of stroke. However, there has been concern regarding the limitations of the Wingspan stent system used in SAMMPRIS and the lack of an angioplasty-only group to assess potential benefit from surgical intervention.[63]

Of note, there was an unexpected reduced rate of stroke and death in the medical management group in the SAMMPRIS trial.[62] In WASID patients treated with aspirin or warfarin had 10.7% 30-day risk of stroke or death (vs 5.8% in SAMMPRIS) and the 1-year rate of the primary end point was 25% (vs 12.2% in SAMMPRIS).[60] The SAMMPRIS authors suggested that this could be related to the use of DAPT, which was supported by the Clopidogrel plus Aspirin for infarction reduction in acute stroke or TIA patients with large artery stenosis and microembolic signals (CLAIR) trial, which demonstrated reduced rates of ipsilateral microemboli in patients with recently symptomatic ICAD treated with DAPT.[64] Patients in the CLAIR trial were randomized to either DAPT with aspirin, 75 to 160 mg daily, plus clopidogrel, 300 mg, on Day 1 followed by 75 mg daily or monotherapy with aspirin, 75 to 160 mg daily, for 1 week.[64,65] The authors of SAMMPRIS ultimately concluded that adding clopidogrel to aspirin for the first 90 days in addition to aggressive management of risk factors was recommended.[62] Further RCTs are necessary to determine whether DAPT is in fact superior to monotherapy for prevention of stroke. In addition, further trials are also necessary to assess the utility of neuroendovascular intervention other than stenting via the wingspan stent and the effects of this therapy in different patient populations with ICAD.

MOYAMOYA DISEASE

Moyamoya disease (MMD) is a chronic occlusive vascular disease that involves progressive stenosis of the intracranial internal carotid arteries and the proximal middle and anterior cerebral arteries leading to collateralization. In one study of adult MMD in China, the posterior cerebral arteries provided collateral flow and were important for maintaining cerebral blood flow.[66] Other authors have noted that the posterior cerebral arteries can become involved in advanced stages of MMD among Asian patients, leading to occlusion and increased risk of recurrent ischemic stroke secondary to reduced collateral flow from leptomeningeal collaterals.[67–69]

With regards to antiplatelet therapy, the guidelines for diagnosis and treatment of MMD in Japan initially recommended antiplatelet therapy because there was no difference in outcome.[70] However, over a longer follow-up interval, surgical revascularization for patients with ischemic symptoms demonstrated improvement in neurologic outcome.[71]

A retrospective cohort study evaluated predictors of recurrent ischemic stroke among Asian adults with MMD who presented with ischemic stroke and received either surgical (indirect encephaloduroarteriosynangiosis) or nonsurgical (antiplatelet) management.[69] Among nonsurgical patients, eight (13.6%) experienced recurrent ischemic stroke during follow-up (mean follow-up, 29 months). Based on the Kaplan-Meier estimate, the risk of recurrent ischemic stroke in nonsurgical patients was only 1.6% in the first year but increased to 11.8% at

5 years. In this group posterior cerebral artery stenosis (defined as >50% stenosis on digital subtraction angiography) and decreased or global decreased cerebral vascular reserve were identified as significant risk factors for recurrent ischemic stroke. The primary treatment modality for patients in the nonsurgical group consisted of antiplatelet monotherapy with either aspirin, clopidogrel, or cilostazol (41 patients; 69.5%), whereas combination therapy with either aspirin and clopidogrel or aspirin and cilostazol was used in 12 patients (20.3%).

Among surgically treated patients, only 12 (26.7%) did not receive any antiplatelet therapy, whereas 30 (66.7%) received single antiplatelet therapy and three (6.7%) received combination antiplatelet therapy. The greatest risk for stroke occurred within the first 30-days following surgery (six patients; 13.3%) with a Kaplan-Meier estimate of 24.4% in the first year, maintained at 24.4% at 5 years. This is in part explained by the time required for surgical collaterals to develop following indirect revascularization.[72,73] Finally, the study by Noh and colleagues[69] also found that diabetes was an independent risk factor for recurrent stroke in both groups, suggesting that the presence of this comorbidity may itself be an indication for medical therapy in addition to surgery if indicated.

STROKE

The 2018 AHA guidelines for AIS recommend initiation of antiplatelet therapy with aspirin within 24 to 48 hours, with delay up to 24 hours in patients who receive intravenous alteplase (COR I, LOE A).[26] A meta-analysis concluded that aspirin (50–150 mg) provides an expected 13% relative risk reduction in serious vascular events,[74] with an expected additional 18% relative risk reduction with the addition of dipyridamole (400 mg/d). For patients presenting with minor stroke, treatment for 21 days with DAPT (aspirin and clopidogrel) initiated within 24 hours may reduce the risk of secondary stroke for up to 90 days from symptom onset.[26] Among patients who experience noncardioembolic AIS while taking aspirin, there is insufficient evidence to recommend increasing aspirin dosage or switching to a different antiplatelet drug for the purpose of secondary stroke prevention (COR IIb, LOE B-R).[26] This is supported by class I evidence from a post hoc analysis of 838 patients from the Secondary Prevention of Small Subcortical Strokes (SPS3) trial, which compared aspirin plus clopidogrel versus aspirin plus placebo in patients who develop a lacunar stroke while taking aspirin.[75] In addition, the authors found that adding clopidogrel increased the risk of major extracranial hemorrhage.[75] The decision to initiate or continue antiplatelet therapy in the setting of hemorrhagic transformation may be considered on a case-by-case basis depending on the clinical indication and a risk-versus-benefit analysis (LOR IIB, LOE B-NR).[26]

Review of key data that influenced the use of antiplatelet therapy in stroke include the International Stroke Trial (IST), a randomized open-label trial that compared aspirin (300 mg daily) and subcutaneous heparin. The results demonstrated a small but significant long-term benefit for the use of aspirin at 6 months.[76] The authors suggested that aspirin should be initiated as soon as possible following the initial AIS, and recommended an initial dose of 300 mg, with possible lower maintenance dose.[76] The Chinese Acute Stroke Trial (CAST) published in the same year was a large randomized placebo-controlled trial that found a significant reduction in mortality and recurrent ischemic stroke with the use of aspirin (160 mg daily) when initiated within 48 hours of AIS.[77]

Clopidogrel Versus Aspirin

The CAPRIE trial was the first blinded long-term RCT to compare the efficacy of clopidogrel (75 mg once daily) with aspirin (325 mg once daily) in prevention of thrombotic events, including ischemic stroke, MI, or vascular death. The study enrolled 19,185 patients with recent ischemic stroke, MI, or symptomatic peripheral arterial disease over a 3-year period. The authors found a statistically significant relative risk reduction of primary outcome (8.7%; $P = .043$) in favor of clopidogrel, without an increased risk of intracranial hemorrhage or gastrointestinal hemorrhage.[26,76] However, among subgroup analyses of stroke and MI, the difference was not significant.[76]

Clopidogrel and Aspirin Versus Clopidogrel

The Management of Atherothrombosis with Clopidogrel in High-risk patients (MATCH) trial was a randomized, double-blind, placebo-controlled trial. It compared clopidogrel alone (75 mg daily) with clopidogrel (75 mg daily) in combination with aspirin (75 mg daily) for the prevention of thrombotic events, vascular death, or rehospitalization for acute ischemic events among patients already taking clopidogrel who had either a recent ischemic stroke or TIA and at least one additional vascular risk factor. The authors found that although there was a 1% absolute risk reduction in the combination group, this was not statistically significant. They concluded that there was no significant long-term benefit to DAPT.[44] Moreover, the authors found an increased risk of life-threatening and major bleeding events among patients treated with DAPT.[44] These findings contrasted with the Clopidogrel in High-risk patients with Acute Nondisabling Cerebrovascular Events (CHANCE) trial, which investigated aspirin alone versus clopidogrel plus aspirin among patients presenting with minor stroke (National Institutes of Health Stroke Scale $\leq$3) or high-risk TIA.[78]

CHANCE was a randomized, double-blind, placebo controlled trial in which all patients received an initial dose of aspirin (75–300 mg) and were started with either a loading dose of clopidogrel (300 mg) followed by 21 days of aspirin (75 mg daily) plus clopidogrel (75 mg daily), then clopidogrel plus placebo until Day 90; or aspirin (75 mg daily) plus placebo for 90 days.[78] The authors concluded that the combination therapy was superior to aspirin alone for reducing the risk of stroke within the first 3 months after initial ischemia when initiated within 24 hours after symptom onset. Moreover, there was no increased risk of hemorrhage.[78] The benefit of early initiation of DAPT was maintained at 1-year follow-up.[79] The primary concern was that this study was carried out among a Chinese population.

Given the findings in CHANCE, the Platelet-Oriented Inhibition in New TIA and Minor Ischemic Stroke (POINT) trial was recently published in 2018 and was aimed to determine the benefit of DAPT to other populations. This study randomly assigned 4881 patients with minor ischemic stroke or high-risk TIA to treatment with either clopidogrel (loading dose 600 mg Day 1, then 75 mg daily) plus aspirin (50–325 mg daily) or aspirin (50–325 mg daily) plus placebo.[80] The trial was stopped early by the data and safety monitoring board after 84% enrollment because of interim analysis demonstrating that clopidogrel plus aspirin was associated with a significantly higher risk of major hemorrhage (0.9% vs 0.4%; hazard ratio [HR], 2.32; $P = .02$) when compared with aspirin monotherapy at 90 days. Nonetheless, the study did find that there was a significantly lower risk of major ischemic events (5.0% vs 6.5%; HR, 0.75; $P = .02$) in the DAPT group versus the aspirin group. Most ischemic events were noted to occur during the first week after the initial episode, and in secondary analysis the benefit of DAPT was greater within the first week and first month than at 90 days following the initial event. The risk for hemorrhage was greater during the period from 8 to 90 days. Of note, both the CHANCE and POINT trials specifically included patients who were not candidates for either intravenous thrombolysis or endovascular thrombectomy (low National Institutes of Health Stroke Scale) and did not have a clear cardioembolic source with planned anticoagulation.

Aspirin and Dipyridamole Versus Aspirin

The European/Australian Stroke Prevention in Reversible Ischemia Trial (ESPRIT) randomly assigned more than 2500 patients to aspirin (30–325 mg daily) with (n = 1363) or without (n = 1376) dipyridamole (200 mg twice daily) within 6 months of TIA or minor stroke. The DAPT group demonstrated a 1% absolute risk reduction of composite primary outcome of vascular mortality, nonfatal stroke, nonfatal MI, or major bleeding compared with patients treated with aspirin alone.[81] A meta-analysis of six trials (n = 7795) comparing aspirin plus dipyridamole versus aspirin alone found that there was a statistically significant 18% lower relative risk of serious vascular event within the combination therapy group versus aspirin alone.[41,74,82–86]

Aspirin and Dipyridamole Versus Clopidogrel

The Prevention Regimen for Effectively Avoiding Second Strokes (PROFESS) trial, included greater than 20,000 patients and compared the efficacy of aspirin, 25 mg daily, in addition to 200 mg extended-release dipyridamole twice a day versus clopidogrel, 75 mg daily, in the prevention of recurrent noncardioembolic stroke.[87] The trial failed to demonstrate noninferiority, and was significantly limited given low statistical power. The authors did find that there were similar rates of recurrent stroke in both groups (HR, 1.03), but that there was an increased risk of major hemorrhagic events in the aspirin/extended-release dipyridamole group versus clopidogrel (HR, 1.15).[87] Despite this, there was not a significant difference in the risk of fatal or disabling strokes between the two groups.

SUMMARY

The role of antiplatelet therapy continues to be of great importance in the treatment of neurosurgical patients, particularly with the expansion of endovascular neurosurgery. There is inadequate evidence to suggest that there is an ideal antiplatelet therapy regimen for each disease process or endovascular intervention. The continued investigation of these drugs and their clinical roles is of the utmost importance now more than ever. Ideally, further studies will aim to address not only the best agents and timing/duration of therapy, but also what other potential antithrombotic mechanisms can be exploited to minimize complications, such as untoward hemorrhage.

REFERENCES

1. Topol EJ, Ferguson JJ, Weisman HF, et al. Long-term protection from myocardial ischemic events in a randomized trial of brief integrin beta3 blockade with percutaneous coronary intervention. EPIC Investigator Group. Evaluation of platelet IIb/IIIa inhibition for prevention of ischemic complication. JAMA 1997;278(6):479–84.
2. Choi HH, Lee JJ, Cho YD, et al. Antiplatelet Premedication for Stent-Assisted Coil Embolization of Intracranial Aneurysms: Low-Dose Prasugrel vs Clopidogrel. Neurosurgery December 2017. https://doi.org/10.1093/neuros/nyx591.
3. Rossen JD, Chalouhi N, Wassef SN, et al. Incidence of cerebral ischemic events after discontinuation of clopidogrel in patients with intracranial aneurysms treated with stent-assisted techniques. J Neurosurg 2012;117(5):929–33.
4. Ryu C-W, Park S, Shin HS, et al. Complications in Stent-Assisted Endovascular Therapy of Ruptured Intracranial Aneurysms and Relevance to Antiplatelet Administration: A Systematic Review. AJNR Am J Neuroradiol 2015;36(9):1682–8.
5. Bhatt DL. Current Role of Platelet Glycoprotein IIb/IIIa Inhibitors in Acute Coronary Syndromes. JAMA 2000;284(12):1549.
6. Kong DF, Califf RM, Miller DP, et al. Clinical outcomes of therapeutic agents that block the platelet glycoprotein IIb/IIIa integrin in ischemic heart disease. Circulation 1998;98(25):2829–35.
7. Lincoff AM, Califf RM, Topol EJ. Platelet glycoprotein IIb/IIIa receptor blockade in coronary artery disease. J Am Coll Cardiol 2000;35(5):1103–15.
8. Antithrombotic Trialists' Collaboration. Collaborative meta-analysis of randomised trials of antiplatelet therapy for prevention of death, myocardial infarction, and stroke in high risk patients. BMJ 2002;324(7329):71–86.
9. Dornbos D 3rd, Katz JS, Youssef P, et al. Glycoprotein IIb/IIIa inhibitors in prevention and rescue treatment of thromboembolic complications during endovascular embolization of intracranial aneurysms. Neurosurgery 2018;82(3):268–77.
10. Skukalek SL, Winkler AM, Kang J, et al. Effect of antiplatelet therapy and platelet function testing on hemorrhagic and thrombotic complications in patients with cerebral aneurysms treated with the pipeline embolization device: a review and meta-analysis. J Neurointerv Surg 2016;8(1):58–65.
11. Becske T, Kallmes DF, Saatci I, et al. Pipeline for uncoilable or failed aneurysms: results from a multicenter clinical trial. Radiology 2013;267(3):858–68.
12. Delgado Almandoz JE, Crandall BM, Scholz JM, et al. Pre-procedure P2Y12 reaction units value predicts perioperative thromboembolic and hemorrhagic complications in patients with cerebral aneurysms treated with the Pipeline Embolization Device. J Neurointerv Surg 2013;5(Suppl 3):iii3–10.
13. Texakalidis P, Bekelis K, Atallah E, et al. Flow diversion with the pipeline embolization device for

patients with intracranial aneurysms and antiplatelet therapy: a systematic literature review. Clin Neurol Neurosurg 2017;161:78–87.

14. Daou B, Starke RM, Chalouhi N, et al. P2Y12 reaction units: effect on hemorrhagic and thromboembolic complications in patients with cerebral aneurysms treated with the pipeline embolization device. Neurosurgery 2016;78(1):27–33.

15. Delgado Almandoz JE, Almandoz JED, Crandall RM, et al. Last-recorded P2Y12 reaction units value is strongly associated with thromboembolic and hemorrhagic complications occurring up to 6 months after treatment in patients with cerebral aneurysms treated with the pipeline embolization device. AJNR Am J Neuroradiol 2013;35(1):128–35.

16. Adeeb N, Griessenauer CJ, Foreman PM, et al. Use of platelet function testing before pipeline embolization device placement: a multicenter cohort study. Stroke 2017;48(5):1322–30.

17. Atallah E, Saad H, Bekelis K, et al. Safety and efficacy of a 600-mg loading dose of clopidogrel 24 hours before pipeline embolization device treatment. World Neurosurg 2017;106:529–35.

18. Tan LA, Keigher KM, Munich SA, et al. Thromboembolic complications with Pipeline Embolization Device placement: impact of procedure time, number of stents and pre-procedure P2Y12 reaction unit (PRU) value. J Neurointerv Surg 2015;7(3):217–21.

19. Patel A, Miller TR, Shivashankar R, et al. Early angiographic signs of acute thrombus formation following cerebral aneurysm treatment with the Pipeline embolization device. J Neurointerv Surg 2017; 9(11):1125–30.

20. Hall R, Mazer CD. Antiplatelet drugs: a review of their pharmacology and management in the perioperative period. Anesth Analg 2011;112(2):292–318.

21. Chalouhi N, Jabbour P, Daou B, et al. A new protocol for anticoagulation with tirofiban during flow diversion. Neurosurgery 2016;78(5):670–4.

22. CADISS trial investigators, Markus HS, Hayter E, Levi C, et al. Antiplatelet treatment compared with anticoagulation treatment for cervical artery dissection (CADISS): a randomised trial. Lancet Neurol 2015;14(4):361–7.

23. Biousse V, D'Anglejan-Chatillon J, Touboul PJ, et al. Time course of symptoms in extracranial carotid artery dissections. A series of 80 patients. Stroke 1995;26(2):235–9.

24. Georgiadis D, Arnold M, von Buedingen HC, et al. Aspirin vs anticoagulation in carotid artery dissection: a study of 298 patients. Neurology 2009; 72(21):1810–5.

25. Debette S, Leys D. Cervical-artery dissections: predisposing factors, diagnosis, and outcome. Lancet Neurol 2009;8(7):668–78.

26. Powers WJ, Rabinstein AA, Ackerson T, et al. 2018 guidelines for the early management of patients with acute ischemic stroke: a guideline for healthcare professionals from the American Heart Association/American Stroke Association. Stroke 2018; 49(3):e46–110.

27. Ricotta JJ, Aburahma A, Ascher E, et al. Updated Society for Vascular Surgery guidelines for management of extracranial carotid disease. J Vasc Surg 2011;54(3):e1–31.

28. Brott TG, Halperin JL, Abbara S, et al. 2011 ASA/ACCF/AHA/AANN/AANS/ACR/ASNR/CNS/SAIP/SCAI/SIR/SNIS/SVM/SVS guideline on the management of patients with extracranial carotid and vertebral artery disease: executive summary: a report of the American College of Cardiology Foundation/American Heart Association Task Force on Practice Guidelines, and the American Stroke Association, American Association of Neuroscience Nurses, American Association of Neurological Surgeons, American College of Radiology, American Society of Neuroradiology, Congress of Neurological Surgeons, Society of Atherosclerosis Imaging and Prevention, Society for Cardiovascular Angiography and Interventions, Society of Interventional Radiology, Society of NeuroInterventional Surgery, Society for Vascular Medicine, and Society for Vascular Surgery. J Am Coll Cardiol 2011;57(8): 1002–44.

29. Paciaroni M, Silvestrelli G, Caso V, et al. Neurovascular territory involved in different etiological subtypes of ischemic stroke in the Perugia Stroke Registry. Eur J Neurol 2003;10(4):361–5.

30. Bogousslavsky J, Van Melle G, Regli F. The Lausanne Stroke Registry: analysis of 1,000 consecutive patients with first stroke. Stroke 1988;19(9):1083–92.

31. Redgrave JN, Rothwell PM. Asymptomatic carotid stenosis: what to do. Curr Opin Neurol 2007;20(1): 58–64.

32. Abbott AL. Medical (nonsurgical) intervention alone is now best for prevention of stroke associated with asymptomatic severe carotid stenosis: results of a systematic review and analysis. Stroke 2009; 40(10):e573–83.

33. Marquardt L, Geraghty OC, Mehta Z, et al. Low risk of ipsilateral stroke in patients with asymptomatic carotid stenosis on best medical treatment: a prospective, population-based study. Stroke 2010; 41(1):e11–7.

34. Woo K, Garg J, Hye RJ, et al. Contemporary results of carotid endarterectomy for asymptomatic carotid stenosis. Stroke 2010;41(5):975–9.

35. Paciaroni M, Bogousslavsky J. Antithrombotic therapy in carotid artery stenosis: an update. Eur Neurol 2015;73(1–2):51–6.

36. Ederle J, Brown MM. The evidence for medicine versus surgery for carotid stenosis. Eur J Radiol 2006;60(1):3–7.

37. Côté R, Battista RN, Abrahamowicz M, et al. Lack of effect of aspirin in asymptomatic patients with

carotid bruits and substantial carotid narrowing. The Asymptomatic Cervical Bruit Study Group. Ann Intern Med 1995;123(9):649–55.

38. Meschia JF, Bushnell C, Boden-Albala B, et al. Guidelines for the primary prevention of stroke. Stroke 2014;45(12):3754–832.

39. Campbell CL, Smyth S, Montalescot G, et al. Aspirin dose for the prevention of cardiovascular disease: a systematic review. JAMA 2007;297(18):2018–24.

40. Lanzino G, Rabinstein AA, Brown RD Jr. Treatment of carotid artery stenosis: medical therapy, surgery, or stenting? Mayo Clin Proc 2009;84(4):362–87 [quiz: 367–8].

41. Bhatt DL, Fox KAA, Hacke W, et al. Clopidogrel and aspirin versus aspirin alone for the prevention of atherothrombotic events. N Engl J Med 2006; 354(16):1706–17.

42. Fox KAA, Mehta SR, Peters R, et al. Benefits and risks of the combination of clopidogrel and aspirin in patients undergoing surgical revascularization for non-ST-elevation acute coronary syndrome: the Clopidogrel in Unstable angina to prevent Recurrent ischemic Events (CURE) Trial. Circulation 2004; 110(10):1202–8.

43. Steinhubl SR, Berger PB, Mann JT 3rd, et al. Early and sustained dual oral antiplatelet therapy following percutaneous coronary intervention: a randomized controlled trial. JAMA 2002;288(19):2411–20.

44. Diener H-C, Bogousslavsky J, Brass LM, et al. Aspirin and clopidogrel compared with clopidogrel alone after recent ischaemic stroke or transient ischaemic attack in high-risk patients (MATCH): randomised, double-blind, placebo-controlled trial. Lancet 2004;364(9431):331–7.

45. The CASANOVA Study Group. Carotid surgery versus medical therapy in asymptomatic carotid stenosis. The CASANOVA Study Group. Stroke 1991; 22(10):1229–35.

46. Touze E. Treatment of carotid stenosis. Curr Vasc Pharmacol 2012;10(6):734–8.

47. Rothwell PM, Giles MF, Chandratheva A, et al. Effect of urgent treatment of transient ischaemic attack and minor stroke on early recurrent stroke (EXPRESS study): a prospective population-based sequential comparison. Lancet 2007;370(9596):1432–42.

48. Sacco RL, Adams R, Albers G, et al. Guidelines for prevention of stroke in patients with ischemic stroke or transient ischemic attack: a statement for healthcare professionals from the American Heart Association/American Stroke Association Council on Stroke: co-sponsored by the Council on Cardiovascular Radiology and Intervention: the American Academy of Neurology affirms the value of this guideline. Stroke 2006;37(2):577–617.

49. Eikelboom JW, Hirsh J. Bleeding and management of bleeding. Eur Heart J Suppl 2006;8(suppl_G): G38–45.

50. Albers GW, Amarenco P, Easton JD, et al. Antithrombotic and thrombolytic therapy for ischemic stroke: American College of Chest Physicians evidence-based clinical practice guidelines (8th Edition). Chest 2008;133(6 Suppl):630S–69S.

51. Wolf PA, Clagett GP, Easton JD, et al. Preventing ischemic stroke in patients with prior stroke and transient ischemic attack: a statement for healthcare professionals from the Stroke Council of the American Heart Association. Stroke 1999;30(9):1991–4.

52. Johnston SC, Nguyen-Huynh MN, Schwarz ME, et al. National Stroke Association guidelines for the management of transient ischemic attacks. Ann Neurol 2006;60(3):301–13.

53. Markus HS, Droste DW, Kaps M, et al. Dual antiplatelet therapy with clopidogrel and aspirin in symptomatic carotid stenosis evaluated using Doppler embolic signal detection: the Clopidogrel and Aspirin for Reduction of Emboli in Symptomatic Carotid Stenosis (CARESS) trial. Circulation 2005; 111(17):2233–40.

54. Enomoto Y, Yoshimura S. Antiplatelet therapy for carotid artery stenting. Interv Neurol 2012;1(3–4):151–63.

55. McKevitt FM, Randall MS, Cleveland TJ, et al. The benefits of combined anti-platelet treatment in carotid artery stenting. Eur J Vasc Endovasc Surg 2005;29(5):522–7.

56. Sacco RL, Kargman DE, Gu Q, et al. Race-ethnicity and determinants of intracranial atherosclerotic cerebral infarction: the Northern Manhattan Stroke Study. Stroke 1995;26(1):14–20.

57. Chimowitz MI, Kokkinos J, Strong J, et al. The warfarin-aspirin symptomatic intracranial disease study. Neurology 1995;45(8):1488–93.

58. Prognosis of patients with symptomatic vertebral or basilar artery stenosis. Stroke 1998;29(7):1389–92.

59. Chimowitz MI, Lynn MJ, Howlett-Smith H, et al. Comparison of warfarin and aspirin for symptomatic intracranial arterial stenosis. N Engl J Med 2005; 352(13):1305–16.

60. Turan TN, Maidan L, Cotsonis G, et al. Failure of antithrombotic therapy and risk of stroke in patients with symptomatic intracranial stenosis. Stroke 2009;40(2):505–9.

61. Kasner SE, Lynn MJ, Chimowitz MI, et al. Warfarin vs aspirin for symptomatic intracranial stenosis: subgroup analyses from WASID. Neurology 2006; 67(7):1275–8.

62. Chimowitz MI, Lynn MJ, Derdeyn CP, et al. Stenting versus aggressive medical therapy for intracranial arterial stenosis. N Engl J Med 2011;365(11):993–1003.

63. Farooq MU, Al-Ali F, Min J, et al. Reviving intracranial angioplasty and stenting "SAMMPRIS and beyond." Front Neurol 2014;5:101.

64. Wong KSL, Chen C, Fu J, et al. Clopidogrel plus aspirin versus aspirin alone for reducing

embolisation in patients with acute symptomatic cerebral or carotid artery stenosis (CLAIR study): a randomised, open-label, blinded-endpoint trial. Lancet Neurol 2010;9(5):489–97.

65. Lau AY, Zhao Y, Chen C, et al. Dual antiplatelets reduce microembolic signals in patients with transient ischemic attack and minor stroke: subgroup analysis of CLAIR study. Int J Stroke 2014;9(Suppl A100):127–32.

66. Bao X-Y, Duan L, Yang W-Z, et al. Clinical features, surgical treatment, and long-term outcome in pediatric patients with moyamoya disease in China. Cerebrovasc Dis 2015;39(2):75–81.

67. Kim J-M, Lee S-H, Roh J-K. Changing ischaemic lesion patterns in adult moyamoya disease. J Neurol Neurosurg Psychiatry 2009;80(1):36–40.

68. Yamada I, Himeno Y, Suzuki S, et al. Posterior circulation in moyamoya disease: angiographic study. Radiology 1995;197(1):239–46.

69. Noh HJ, Kim SJ, Kim JS, et al. Long term outcome and predictors of ischemic stroke recurrence in adult moyamoya disease. J Neurol Sci 2015;359(1–2):381–8.

70. Fukui M. Guidelines for the diagnosis and treatment of spontaneous occlusion of the circle of Willis ('moyamoya' disease). Research Committee on Spontaneous Occlusion of the Circle of Willis (Moyamoya Disease) of the Ministry of Health and Welfare, Japan. Clin Neurol Neurosurg 1997;99(Suppl 2): S238–40.

71. Yamada S, Oki K, Itoh Y, et al. Effects of surgery and antiplatelet therapy in ten-year follow-up from the registry Study of Research Committee on Moyamoya Disease in Japan. J Stroke Cerebrovasc Dis 2016; 25(2):340–9.

72. Houkin K, Kuroda S, Ishikawa T, et al. Neovascularization (angiogenesis) after revascularization in moyamoya disease. Which technique is most useful for moyamoya disease? Acta Neurochir 2000; 142(3):269–76.

73. Houkin K, Nakayama N, Kuroda S, et al. How does angiogenesis develop in pediatric moyamoya disease after surgery? A prospective study with MR angiography. Childs Nerv Syst 2004;20(10):734–41.

74. O'Donnell MJ, Hankey GJ, Eikelboom JW. Antiplatelet therapy for secondary prevention of noncardioembolic ischemic stroke: a critical review. Stroke 2008;39(5):1638–46.

75. Côté R, Zhang Y, Hart RG, et al. ASA failure: does the combination ASA/clopidogrel confer better long-term vascular protection? Neurology 2014; 82(5):382–9.

76. CAPRIE Steering Committee. A randomised, blinded, trial of clopidogrel versus aspirin in patients at risk of ischaemic events (CAPRIE). CAPRIE Steering Committee. Lancet 1996;348(9038):1329–39.

77. CAST: randomised placebo-controlled trial of early aspirin use in 20,000 patients with acute ischaemic stroke. CAST (Chinese Acute Stroke Trial) Collaborative Group. Lancet 1997;349(9066):1641–9.

78. Wang Y, Wang Y, Zhao X, et al. Clopidogrel with aspirin in acute minor stroke or transient ischemic attack. N Engl J Med 2013;369(1):11–9.

79. Wang Y, Pan Y, Zhao X, et al. Clopidogrel with aspirin in acute minor stroke or transient ischemic attack (CHANCE) trial: one-year outcomes. Circulation 2015;132(1):40–6.

80. Johnston SC, Easton JD, Farrant M, et al. Clopidogrel and aspirin in acute ischemic stroke and high-risk TIA. N Engl J Med 2018. https://doi.org/10.1056/NEJMoa1800410.

81. ESPRIT Study Group, Halkes PHA, van Gijn J, et al. Aspirin plus dipyridamole versus aspirin alone after cerebral ischaemia of arterial origin (ESPRIT): randomised controlled trial. Lancet 2006;367(9523): 1665–73.

82. Bousser MG, Eschwege E, Haguenau M, et al. "AICLA" controlled trial of aspirin and dipyridamole in the secondary prevention of athero-thrombotic cerebral ischemia. Stroke 1983;14(1):5–14.

83. Diener HC, Cunha L, Forbes C, et al. European Stroke Prevention Study 2. Dipyridamole and acetylsalicylic acid in the secondary prevention of stroke. J Neurol Sci 1996;143(1–2):1–13.

84. Guiraud-Chaumeil B, Rascol A, David J, et al. Prevention of recurrences of cerebral ischemic vascular accidents by platelet antiaggregants. Results of a 3-year controlled therapeutic trial. Rev Neurol 1982; 138(5):367–85 [in French].

85. Persantine Aspirin Trial in cerebral ischemia. Part II: endpoint results. The American-Canadian Co-Operative Study group. Stroke 1985;16(3):406–15.

86. Bhatt DL, Flather MD, Hacke W, et al. Patients with prior myocardial infarction, stroke, or symptomatic peripheral arterial disease in the CHARISMA trial. J Am Coll Cardiol 2007;49(19):1982–8.

87. Sacco RL, Diener H-C, Yusuf S, et al. Aspirin and extended-release dipyridamole versus clopidogrel for recurrent stroke. N Engl J Med 2008;359(12): 1238–51.

Common Conditions Requiring Long-Term Anticoagulation in Neurosurgical Patients

Augustus J. Perez, MD[a], Gerald A. Grant, MD[b],*

KEYWORDS

- Anticoagulation • Antithrombotic • Thrombophilia • Prothrombotic • Thrombogenic
- Atrial fibrillation • Mechanical heart valve • Bioprosthetic valve

KEY POINTS

- Atrial fibrillation, mechanical heart valves, and thrombophilia represent chronic medical conditions requiring anticoagulation.
- Warfarin has represented the standard treatment of these conditions.
- Although direct oral anticoagulants have shown promise and have antidotes to immediately reverse their activity, studies have not demonstrated universal efficacy.
- Chronic anticoagulation in neurosurgical patients must be approached by taking into account both the scientific literature supporting its use with individual patient profiles.

INTRODUCTION

Long-term anticoagulant therapy serves primarily to arrest the propagation of thrombus, thereby preventing the development of highly morbid conditions related to impairment of vital tissues at the terminus of the vascular bed. Costly sequelae can include cerebral ischemia, pulmonary embolism (PE) and infarct, and compromise or loss of limbs. The use of anticoagulation in neurosurgical patients urges a continued risk analysis by the surgeon given the inherent complexity proffered by this clinicopathologic schema in the setting of thrombophilia. Therefore, management of neurosurgical patients with conditions such as atrial fibrillation (AF), mechanical heart valves, and other prothrombotic states necessitates application of a vetted strategy to mitigate the potential complications of anticoagulation.

With their continued development, the direct oral anticoagulants (DOACs), which include the direct thrombin and factor X inhibitors, have become de rigueur in the management of certain subsets of this patient population. Their use in neurosurgical patients yields new considerations to be had, in particular, the introduction of adequate reversal agents. Previously, idarucizumab (or Praxbind) was the only reversal agent against dabigatran (Pradaxa) approved by the Food and Drug Administration (FDA). At the time of drafting this article, the FDA released its approval of andexanet alfa (AndexXa) for use against apixaban (Eliquis) and rivaroxaban (Xarelto). Further enumeration of these considerations

Disclosure Statement: The authors have nothing to disclose.
[a] Pediatric Neurosurgery, Department of Neurosurgery, Stanford University Medical Center, 300 Pasteur Drive Room R211, MC 5325, Stanford, CA 94305, USA; [b] Department of Neurosurgery, Stanford University Medical Center, 300 Pasteur Drive Room R211, MC 5327, Stanford, CA 94305, USA
* Corresponding author.
E-mail address: ggrant2@stanford.edu

Neurosurg Clin N Am 29 (2018) 529–535
https://doi.org/10.1016/j.nec.2018.06.009
1042-3680/18/© 2018 Elsevier Inc. All rights reserved.

relates to patient management and clinical trajectory regarding secondary hemorrhage potential.

This article serves as a brief exposition of the more common chronic clinical entities that require the use of prolonged anticoagulant therapy with special consideration for neurosurgical patients. This exposition includes a discussion of established treatment strategies across all available treatment options.

THROMBOEMBOLIC RISK ASSESSMENT AND MANAGEMENT IN ATRIAL FIBRILLATION

With evidence that suggests an increasing incidence and prevalence, AF represents a global health concern that portends a higher consequent risk of death, heart failure, and thromboembolic events.[1–3] As the most common sustained cardiac arrhythmia, the number of individuals worldwide with AF has been estimated at approximately 33.5 million in 2010[3] and the total estimated cost is approximately 1% of health care expenditure.[2] In the United States, the prevalence of AF in 2005 was 3.03 million with a projected increase to 7.56 million by 2050.[4] The Framingham Heart Study provided a lifetime risk of the development of AF as 26% for men and 23% for women aged 40 to 95 years.[5] AF has been historically characterized as occupying a spectrum that ranges from paroxysmal, persistent, long-standing persistent to permanent.

Management of patients with AF focuses on the prevention of the primary sequelae of AF, namely, ischemic stroke secondary to thromboembolism.

However, thromboembolic events can also occur in the systemic and pulmonary circulations. Moreover, stroke and transient ischemic attack (TIA) events in the setting of AF have an augmented severity and have been shown to relate worse outcomes compared with these events in the absence of AF. A study by Anderson and colleagues[6] demonstrated a markedly increased ratio of hemispheric to retinal events in the setting of AF versus carotid disease (25:1 compared with 2:1). AF-related stroke, when compared with stroke without AF, seems to confer increased disability and a higher mortality.[7] Additionally, TIAs with their cause in AF are typically prolonged and associated with MRI diffusion changes. Therefore, the American Heart Association (AHA) revised the stroke definition attempts to reclassify these TIAs as stroke.[8]

Current Methods in Risk Assessment

Estimating embolic risk becomes crucial for patient management and, in conjunction with annualized rates of hemorrhagic complications, is the pivot point for decisions on prescribing anticoagulation therapy. Tools, including the one outlined later, have long been in development to navigate this scenario; but a foray into the nuances of this judgment pathway is, of course, beyond the scope of this article. **Table 1** outlines the CHA_2DS_2-VASc model, the contemporary risk assessment model. The resultant score ranges from 0 to a maximum of 9 and represents a range of stroke risk with mean rates of stroke starting at 0.2, 0.6, and 2.2 for scores of 0, 1, and 2, respectively. Most

Table 1
CHA_2DS_2-VASc embolic stroke risk stratification for patients with nonvalvular atrial fibrillation

Definition	Score	Cumulative Score	Unadjusted Ischemic Stroke Rate (% Per Year)
—	—	0	0.2%
Congestive heart failure	1	1	0.6
Hypertension	1	2	2.2
Age ≥75 y old	2	3	3.2
Diabetes mellitus	1	4	4.8
Stroke/TIA/TE	2	5	7.2
Vascular disease (prior MI, PAD, or aortic plaque)	1	6	9.7
Age 65–74 y old	1	7	11.2
Sex category (female)	1	8	10.8
Maximum	*9*	*9*	*12.2*

Abbreviations: MI, myocardial infarction; PAD, peripheral artery disease; TE, thromboembolism.
Modified from Lip GYH, Nieuwlaat R, Pisters R, et al. Refining clinical risk stratification for predicting stroke and thromboembolism in atrial fibrillation using a novel risk factor-based approach: the Euro heart survey on atrial fibrillation. Chest 2010;137(2):266; with permission.

evidence suggests that initiating oral anticoagulation is prudent at scores of 2 or greater.[9–12]

For anticoagulated patients, the observed rate of intracranial hemorrhage (ICH) from the modern literature ranges from 0.2 to 0.4% per year. In 2007, Fang and colleagues[13] demonstrated a rate of ICH and major extracranial hemorrhage of 72 and 98 per 15,300 person-years, respectively. This rate increases in the setting of thrombocytopenia or known coagulation defects, active bleeding or surgery with concern for active bleeding, prior severe bleeding while on oral anticoagulation, suspected aortic dissection, malignant hypertension, and combined use of anticoagulation or antiplatelet agents. Bleeding risk models, such as the HAS-BLED score (Hypertension, Abnormal renal and liver function, Stroke, Bleeding, Labile INR, Elderly, Drugs/Alcohol), have been proposed for anticoagulated patients, but have been met with some contention.[14]

The final algorithm for therapeutic decision making in patients with AF must necessarily be a composite of individualized assessment and utilization of these well-established tools.

Use of Novel Anticoagulation Agents in Atrial Fibrillation

For those patients with nonvalvular AF, the FDA has approved the direct thrombin inhibitor, dabigatran, as well as the factor Xa inhibitors rivaroxaban and apixaban expressly for the prevention of stroke. The Randomized Evaluation of Long-Term Anticoagulation Therapy (RE-LY), Rivaroxaban Once Daily Oral Direct Factor Xa Inhibition Compared with Vitamin K Antagonism for Prevention of Stroke and Embolism Trial in Atrial Fibrillation (ROCKET-AF), and Apixaban for Reduction in Stroke and Other Thromboembolic Events in Atrial Fibrillation (ARISTOTLE) trials, respectively, demonstrated increased rates of stroke prevention or noninferiority to warfarin with an overall decreased risk of major bleeding events. Specifically, all 3 agents were shown to have significantly lower rates of cerebral hemorrhage compared with warfarin.[15–17]

For neurosurgical patients, several questions arise if they are prescribed DOAC.s As mentioned, most of these questions mirror concerns raised with warfarin use and depend on reversal potential. The practitioner will need to weigh several variables that include (a) appropriate timing for restarting anticoagulation in the postoperative period; (b) appropriate timing for restarting anticoagulation in the nonoperative setting, for example, trauma or prior hemorrhage event; (c) determination of mobilization and therapy potential given the likelihood of fall risk; and (d) management of temporary catheters or drains.

MANAGEMENT OF PATIENTS WITH VALVULAR PROSTHESES

Current estimates of the prevalence of valvular heart disease range from 0.02% in those patients less than 45 years old to 9.3% in elderly patients greater than 75 years old.[18] An impressive body of work exists for the surgical treatment of valvulopathy as is evident by the number of prosthetic valves that are or have been available. These prostheses can be categorized as either mechanical (bileaflet, St. Jude Medical Inc, Saint Paul, MN; On-X, CryoLife Inc, Kennesaw, GA; or single-tilting disc) or bioprosthetic (pericardial or allograft porcine, bovine, equine), and selection depends on a variety of clinical factors.

Valvular replacement is not without complication, the most frequent of which are thromboembolic events, namely, cerebrovascular accident, and anticoagulant therapy–related complications for mechanical valves, with bioprosthetic valves having a lower thromboembolic risk profile. Indeed, the observed rate of major embolic events in patients with mechanical valve prostheses not treated with antithrombotic therapy was shown at 4 per 100 patient-years. The risk of thromboembolic stroke in patients with bioprosthetic valves ranges from 0.2% to 3.3% per year.[19–21] Initiation of anticoagulation in patients with valve replacement is dictated by the type of valve and the associated thrombogenicity, the site of valve placement (ie, aortic or mitral), and the presence of comorbid conditions promoting thrombogenesis.

Therapy Recommendations

Contemporary recommendations for anticoagulation goals in patients with valve replacements are derived in large part from the AHA/American College of Cardiology's (ACC) 2014 valve guidelines. These guidelines were updated in 2017. They use a model of target international normalized ratios (INRs) with an acceptable positive or negative margin in lieu of value ranges.[22]

Summary recommendations include the use of vitamin K antagonists (VKAs), for example, warfarin, dosed to the desired target with concomitant use of daily aspirin, especially in patients with mechanical valves. Supplemental recommendations include use of bridging therapy in the immediate postoperative period when deemed appropriate vis-à-vis the risk of hemorrhage. The therapeutic approach varies, and a consensus has yet to be seen. Current strategies include intravenous or subcutaneous unfractionated heparin (UFH) or subcutaneous low-molecular-weight heparin (LMWH) at either prophylactic or therapeutic doses for a period of at least 5 days.

The use of DOACs is not recommended in patients with mechanical valves as demonstrated by the Randomized, Phase II Study to Evaluate the Safety and Pharmacokinetics of Oral Dabigatran Etexilate in Patients after Heart Valve Replacement (RE-ALIGN) trial[23]; evidence is limited for their use in patients with bioprosthetic valves.

Therapeutic goals vary based on the thrombogenicity of the implant. **Table 2** summarizes these goals for specific clinical subsets. For patients with mechanical prosthetic mitral or tricuspid valves without any other risk factors for thromboembolism, the recommended target INR is 3. This same target applies to patients with aortic valves in the setting of additional thromboembolic risk factors, which include AF, previous thromboembolism, left ventricular systolic dysfunction, or a hypercoagulable condition, as well as those patients with older-generation aortic valve prostheses (see **Table 2**). A target INR of 2.5 is desired for current-generation aortic valves in the absence of additional thromboembolic risk factors. For patients with the On-X bileaflet aortic prosthesis and no other thromboembolic risk factors, the INR target is 2 to 3 for the first 3 months after implantation, with the target reduced to 1.5 to 2.0 thereafter.

The treatment strategy for patients with bioprosthetic valves is distinct from those guidelines for mechanical prostheses.[24] For aortic or mitral bioprostheses, treatment with a VKA to a target INR of 2.5 for 3 to 6 months is recommended in conjunction with long-standing aspirin at a dosage of 75 to 100 mg per day. For those patients with additional thromboembolic risk factors, early bridging therapy after implantation is recommended. The use of DOACs for chronic management in valve prostheses has yet to achieve consensus and is not standard practice.

The risk of thromboembolism in these patients must be juxtaposed to the likelihood of major hemorrhagic events, as the latter will have enhanced consequence in neurosurgical patients. Current estimates place the risk of ICH or spinal hemorrhage at 0.57 per 100 patient-years in patients with mechanical valves taking oral anticoagulation. The significant extracranial bleeding risk was 2.1 per 100 patient-years in this same study.[25] The decision for implementation or reimplementation of antithrombotic therapy should be analyzed in light of this risk.

Cause of and Considerations for the Thrombophilic State

The thrombophilic state is determined by those conditions, classified as either acquired or inherited, that subscribe either partially or in totality to the Virchow paradigm: hypercoagulability, endothelial injury, and stasis of blood flow.[26] A synopsis of these conditions is laid out in **Box 1**. In reality, the delineation between acquired and inherited conditions is not steadfast, as multiple risk factors are often identified in patients from either of the two major categories.

Patients at risk will present with superficial venous thrombosis (SVT), deep venous thrombosis (DVT), or PE. These diagnoses are nonexclusionary and progressive: the prevalence of DVT and PE in patients with known SVT has been documented as high as 18% and 7%, respectively.[27]

Table 2
Summary of therapeutic goals for anticoagulation in patients with mechanical valve prostheses

Therapeutic goals for various mechanical valve types	
Following valve placement, 5 d of bridging tx with UFH, LMWH	
Concomitant use of aspirin, 75–100 mg/d	
Valve characteristic	**Therapeutic goal**
Tricuspid valve	Anticoagulation with VKA to goal INR of 3
Mitral valve (including On-X)	
Aortic valve (other than On-X) + *additional thromboembolic risk factors*[a]	
Older-generation aortic valve (eg, ball-in-cage)	
Bileaflet aortic valve (other than On-X)	Anticoagulation with VKA to goal INR of 2.5
Current-generation single-tilting disc aortic valve	
On-X bileaflet aortic valve	Anticoagulation with VKA to goal INR 2–3 for 3 mo, then goal 1.5–2.0

INR values are targets of therapy with permissible margins of 0.5 in either direction based on the model in the AHA/ACC's 2014 valve guidelines.
[a] Including AF, previous thromboembolism, left ventricular systolic dysfunction, or hypercoagulable condition.

Box 1
Risk factors for the development of venous thrombosis

- Hormone replacement therapy
- Other cancer therapies (eg, tamoxifen, thalidomide, lenalidomide)
- Mixed
  - Low protein S levels
  - High factors VIII, IX, XI
  - Hyperhomocysteinemia

Data from Lijfering WM, Rosendaal FR, Cannegieter SC. Risk factors for venous thrombosis - current understanding from an epidemiological point of view. Br J Haematol 2010;149(6):824–33.

Inherited Risk Factors

More than half of all cases of an inherited, or primary, hypercoagulable state are constituted by a factor V Leiden (FVL) or prothrombin gene mutation. In FVL, all forms of coagulation factor V become incapable of responding to activated protein C due to a factor mutation, which confers an increased risk of venous thromboembolism (VTE). This risk has been characterized as a relative risk of 7 in the case of a heterozygous mutation and 80 in the case of a homozygous mutation.[28]

Prothrombin is a vitamin K–dependent protein whose activated derivative, thrombin, is essential in the cleavage of fibrinogen to fibrin, in addition to several other downstream cascade moieties promoting hemostasis. Several polymorphisms of the prothrombin gene product exist, but the most commonly known occurs with a substitution of adenine for guanine at position 20,210 in a noncoding region of the gene. The resulting phenotype manifests as a 30% increase in circulating prothrombin levels relative to controls.[29] The exact mechanism underlying the provision of hypercoagulability in this situation has yet to be elucidated. Compared with the normal population, the prothrombin G20210 A mutation is associated with a 2.8-fold increased likelihood of VTE.[28]

Additional conditions have been posited within the framework of hypercoagulability; however, their role in the generation of a prothrombotic state is unclear. These conditions include heparin cofactor II deficiency, plasminogen deficiency, dysfibrinogenemia, and factor XII deficiency.

Acquired Risk Factors

The most commonly seen acquired factors conferring hypercoagulability are outlined in **Box 1**. It should be noted that these conditions, or at least their resultant states, are conjunctive. A large population-based analysis delineated the 6 most prevalent preexisting medical characteristics of the study cohort, which included (1) more than 48 hours of immobility in the preceding month (45%), (2) hospital admission in the past 3 months (39%), (3) surgery in the past 3 months (34%), (4) malignancy in the past 3 months (34%), (5) infection in the past 3 months (34%), and (6) current hospitalization (26%). Eleven percent (11%) of all VTE episodes had none of these characteristics present at the time of diagnosis, whereas 53% had at least 3.[30]

Of additional interest may be the anatomic risk factors for the development of VTE, specifically DVT. These risk factors have no known genetic component and include

- *Paget-Schroetter syndrome*: a compressive anomaly at the thoracic outlet, typically by the clavicle, cervical rib, or scalenus muscle that predisposes to spontaneous upper extremity venous thrombosis
- *May-Thurner syndrome* (or iliac vein compression syndrome): results from compression of the left common iliac vein by the right common iliac artery against the underlying vertebral body
- *Abnormalities of the inferior vena cava*: agenesis, hypoplasia, or malformation that can lead to recurrent or bilateral lower extremity DVTs in younger patients.[31–34]

SUMMARY

Individualized and focused care is the sine qua non in the philosophy of precision medicine in the current era. Management of those patients with acquired or inherited thrombophilic states, such as AF, valvular prostheses, and other prothrombotic conditions, is no exception to this philosophy. The potential for neurosurgical pathology presents a specific clinical dilemma, as the practitioner constantly treads the precarious and dynamic duality of benefit and consequence engendered by long-term anticoagulation therapy. Strides in preventing thromboembolic events are offset by the risk of significant hemorrhagic complications. Therefore, a unique and evolving treatment plan is required for every patient as one accounts for the global clinical picture. Application of this kind of approach ensures promotion of the best possible outcomes in our patients.

This approach is best exemplified by the advent of the direct anticoagulants. The development and vetting of viable reversal options will dictate the applicability of DOACs to neurosurgical patients, and more widespread adoption of these novel agents will depend on the evolution of their utilization in the setting of discrete clinical and perioperative parameters.

REFERENCES

1. Lip GY, Brechin CM, Lane DA. The global burden of atrial fibrillation and stroke: a systematic review of the epidemiology of atrial fibrillation in regions outside North America and Europe. Chest 2012; 142:1489.

2. Ball J, Carrington MJ, McMurray JJ, et al. Atrial fibrillation: profile and burden of an evolving epidemic in the 21st century. Int J Cardiol 2013;167:1807.

3. Chugh SS, Havmoeller R, Narayanan K, et al. Worldwide epidemiology of atrial fibrillation: a Global Burden of Disease 2010 Study. Circulation 2014; 129:837.

4. Naccarelli GV, Varker H, Lin J, et al. Increasing prevalence of atrial fibrillation and flutter in the United States. Am J Cardiol 2009;104:1534.

5. Lloyd-Jones DM, Wang TJ, Leip EP, et al. Lifetime risk for development of atrial fibrillation: the Framingham Heart Study. Circulation 2004;110:1042.

6. Anderson DC, Kappelle LJ, Eliasziw M, et al. Occurrence of hemispheric and retinal ischemia in atrial fibrillation compared with carotid stenosis. Stroke 2002;33:1963.

7. Lamassa M, Di Carlo A, Pracucci G, et al. Characteristics, outcome, and care of stroke associated with atrial fibrillation in Europe: data from a multicenter multinational hospital-based registry (The European Community Stroke Project). Stroke 2001;32:392.

8. Easton JD, Saver JL, Albers GW, et al. Definition and evaluation of transient ischemic attack: a scientific statement for healthcare professionals from the American Heart Association/American Stroke Association Stroke Council; Council on Cardiovascular Surgery and Anesthesia; Council on Cardiovascular Radiology and Intervention; Council on Cardiovascular Nursing; and the Interdisciplinary Council on Peripheral Vascular Disease. The American Academy of Neurology affirms the value of this statement as an educational tool for neurologists. Stroke 2009; 40:2276.

9. Friberg L, Rosenqvist M, Lip GY. Net clinical benefit of warfarin in patients with atrial fibrillation: a report from the Swedish atrial fibrillation cohort study. Circulation 2012;125:2298.

10. Singer DE, Chang Y, Fang MC, et al. The net clinical benefit of warfarin anticoagulation in atrial fibrillation. Ann Intern Med 2009;151:297.

11. Olesen JB, Lip GY, Lindhardsen J, et al. Risks of thromboembolism and bleeding with thromboprophylaxis in patients with atrial fibrillation: a net clinical benefit analysis using a 'real world' nationwide cohort study. Thromb Haemost 2011; 106:739.

12. Banerjee A, Lane DA, Torp-Pedersen C, et al. Net clinical benefit of new oral anticoagulants (dabigatran, rivaroxaban, apixaban) versus no treatment in a 'real world' atrial fibrillation population: a modelling analysis based on a nationwide cohort study. Thromb Haemost 2012;107:584.

13. Fang MC, Go AS, Chang Y, et al. Death and disability from warfarin-associated intracranial and extracranial hemorrhages. Am J Med 2007;120:700.

14. Lip GY. Implications of the CHA2DS2-VASc and HAS-BLED Scores for thromboprophylaxis in atrial fibrillation. Am J Med 2011;124:111.

15. Connolly SJ, Ezekowitz MD, Yusuf S, et al. Dabigatran versus warfarin in patients with atrial fibrillation. N Engl J Med 2009;361:1139.

16. Patel MR, Mahaffey KW, Garg J, et al. Rivaroxaban versus warfarin in nonvalvular atrial fibrillation. N Engl J Med 2011;365:883.

17. Granger CB, Alexander JH, McMurray JJ, et al. Apixaban versus warfarin in patients with atrial fibrillation. N Engl J Med 2011;365:981.

18. Nkomo VT, Gardin JM, Skelton TN, et al. Burden of valvular heart diseases: a population-based study. Lancet 2006;368:1005.

19. Cannegieter SC, Rosendaal FR, Briët E. Thromboembolic and bleeding complications in patients with mechanical heart valve prostheses. Circulation 1994;89:635.

20. Whitlock RP, Sun JC, Fremes SE, et al. Antithrombotic and thrombolytic therapy for valvular disease: antithrombotic therapy and prevention of thrombosis, 9th ed: American College of Chest Physicians Evidence-Based Clinical Practice Guidelines. Chest 2012;141:e576S.

21. Heras M, Chesebro JH, Fuster V, et al. High risk of thromboemboli early after bioprosthetic cardiac valve replacement. J Am Coll Cardiol 1995;25:1111.

22. Nishimura RA, Otto CM, Bonow RO, et al. 2014 AHA/ACC guideline for the management of patients with valvular heart disease: a report of the American College of Cardiology/American Heart Association Task Force on Practice Guidelines. J Am Coll Cardiol 2014;63:e57.

23. Eikelboom JW, Connolly SJ, Brueckmann M, et al. Dabigatran versus warfarin in patients with mechanical heart valves. N Engl J Med 2013;369: 1206.

24. Nishimura RA, Otto CM, Bonow RO, et al. 2017 AHA/ACC focused update of the 2014 AHA/ACC guideline for the management of patients with valvular heart disease: a report of the American College of Cardiology/American Heart Association Task Force on Clinical Practice Guidelines. J Am Coll Cardiol 2017;70(2):252–89.

25. Cannegieter SC, Rosendaal FR, Wintzen AR, et al. Optimal oral anticoagulant therapy in patients with mechanical heart valves. N Engl J Med 1995;333:11.

26. Virchow R. "Thrombose und Embolie. Gefässentzündung und septische Infektion". Gesammelte Abhandlungen zur wissenschaftlichen Medicin [in German]. Frankfurt am Main: Von Meidinger & Sohn. 1856. p. 219–732. Matzdorff AC, Bell WR. Thrombosis and embolie (1846-1856). Canton (MA): Science History Publications; 1998.

27. Di Minno MN, Ambrosino P, Ambrosini F, et al. Prevalence of deep vein thrombosis and pulmonary embolism in patients with superficial vein thrombosis: a systematic review and meta-analysis. J Thromb Haemost 2016;14:964.

28. Bauer KA. The thrombophilias: well-defined risk factors with uncertain therapeutic implications. Ann Intern Med 2001;135(5):367–73.

29. Poort SR, Rosendaal FR, Reitsma PH, et al. A common genetic variation in the 3'-untranslated region of the prothrombin gene is associated with elevated plasma prothrombin levels and an increase in venous thrombosis. Blood 1996;88:3698.

30. Spencer FA, Emery C, Lessard D, et al. The Worcester Venous Thromboembolism study: a population-based study of the clinical epidemiology of venous thromboembolism. J Gen Intern Med 2006;21:722.

31. Kibbe MR, Ujiki M, Goodwin AL, et al. Iliac vein compression in an asymptomatic patient population. J Vasc Surg 2004;39:937.

32. Chee YL, Culligan DJ, Watson HG. Inferior vena cava malformation as a risk factor for deep venous thrombosis in the young. Br J Haematol 2001;114:878.

33. Ruggeri M, Tosetto A, Castaman G, et al. Congenital absence of the inferior vena cava: a rare risk factor for idiopathic deep-vein thrombosis. Lancet 2001; 357:441.

34. Hamoud S, Nitecky S, Engel A, et al. Hypoplasia of the inferior vena cava with azygous continuation presenting as recurrent leg deep vein thrombosis. Am J Med Sci 2000;319:414.

Reversal of Systemic Anticoagulants and Antiplatelet Therapeutics

David Dornbos III, MD, Shahid M. Nimjee, MD, PhD*

KEYWORDS

- Anti-platelet • Anticoagulation • Stroke • Intracranial hemorrhage

KEY POINTS

- No reversal agents exist for antiplatelet medications, although platelet transfusion and desmopressin administration may partially restore appropriate thrombogenesis.
- Anticoagulation with warfarin is frequently encountered in neurosurgery patients but can be quickly reversed with prothrombin complex concentrate, fresh frozen plasma, or and vitamin K.
- New agents like andexanet alfa and idarucizumab provide reversal strategies for factor Xa inhibitors and direct thrombin inhibitors, respectively.

INTRODUCTION

Coagulopathy secondary to antiplatelet medications and anticoagulation is a frequently encountered source of morbidity in neurosurgical patients. Reversal of these agents plays an important role, whether preparing for elective surgery or in an emergent fashion after trauma or spontaneous intracranial hemorrhage (ICH). Patients treated with anticoagulation carry an annual systemic bleeding incidence of 15% to 20%, with a 2% risk of ICH.[1] Furthermore, 15% of all ICH occurs secondary to anticoagulation treatment[2] and is associated with a substantial mortality of 70%.[3] Despite the utilization of reversal agents or protocols for the majority of current anticoagulants, potential delays in medication reversal can have significant consequences secondary to hematoma expansion.

The advent of newer-generation anticoagulants and antiplatelet agents presents unique challenges. The introduction of new reversal agents for factor Xa inhibitors and direct thrombin inhibitors (DTIs) over the past few years has had a profound effect, showing significant benefit compared with prior reversal protocols. Furthermore, continued development of new antiplatelet agents has presented challenges to limit hemorrhage propagation when a true reversal agent does not exist.

Hemostasis is a dynamic process involving platelet adhesion and aggregation, in addition to the interactions of numerous factors within the coagulation cascade. The intrinsic and extrinsic pathways provide a target for the majority of anticoagulant therapeutics. Contained entirely within the intravascular space, the intrinsic pathway involves the activation of factors XII, XI, and IX in succession, ultimately activating factor Xa with the cofactor XIIIa.[4] The extrinsic pathway, initiated outside of the intravascular space, is initiated by the activation and coassociation of factor VII and tissue factor. The tissue factor VIIa complex with cofactor VIIIa is able to activate factor Xa as the 2 pathways converge. Once activated, factor Xa and cofactor Va convert prothrombin (factor II) to

Disclosure Statement: The authors have nothing to disclose.

Department of Neurological Surgery, Ohio State University Medical Center, N-1014 Doan Hall, 410 West 10th Avenue, Columbus, OH, USA

* Corresponding author.

E-mail address: shahid.nimjee@osumc.edu

thrombin (factor IIa), which then converts fibrinogen to fibrin.[4]

Although the activation of thrombin and fibrin is essential to hemostasis, platelet activation and aggregation are critical to thrombus plug formation. Inactivated platelets contact and bind von Willebrand factor (vWF) at a site of vascular injury via the platelet surface glycoprotein (GP) Ib-IX-V.[5] The small amount of thrombin, generated through the extrinsic pathway at the site of vascular injury, then plays a major role in further thrombus propagation. First, thrombin converts GP IIb/IIIa from a quiescent protein to an active platelet-surface molecule. GP IIb/IIIa then is able to bind fibrin and assist in platelet cross-linking, and it triggers more GP IIb/IIIa molecules to be expressed at the cell surface. Second, thrombin further activates factor VIIIa and Va on the platelet surface, substantially increasing thrombin generation via the coagulation cascades. Finally, thrombin activates factor XIIIa, which is responsible for stabilizing platelet-platelet interactions by cross-linking fibrin monomers.

A thorough understanding of the platelet biology and coagulation underlying hemostasis is vital to the reversal strategies designed to combat coagulation and platelet inhibition in clinical practice. Although many antiplatelet and anticoagulant agents have existed for years, newer agents have posed new challenges. Appropriate reversal strategies for these medications are a vital resource to the neurosurgical armamentarium in combatting medication-induced coagulopathy. This review highlights recent data to provide a comprehensive summary of the latest antiplatelet and anticoagulant therapies and the role of emergency reversal in the setting of ICH or emergent neurosurgical procedures.

ANTIPLATELET AGENTS
Cyclooxygenase Inhibitors

Acetylsalicylic acid (aspirin), with a half-life 30 minutes, is a cyclooxygenase (COX)-1 inhibitor, preventing the metabolism of arachidonic acid and the generation of prostaglandin H2, a precursor to thromboxane A2. Thromboxane A2, after binding to its receptor, induces a significant increase in intracellular calcium, promoting platelet activation and aggregation and creating a substantially prothrombotic environment. Aspirin irreversibly binds to COX-1, effectively inhibiting thromboxane A2 production for the life of the platelet. Additionally, inhibition of COX-1 and COX-2 blocks prostaglandin production, resulting in analgesic and antipyretic effects as well.

Aspirin is an oral medication and is prescribed at a dosage of 81 mg to 325 mg daily. Aspirin is widely used in primary and secondary prevention of ischemic stroke and cardiovascular events, providing a 22% reduction in nonfatal myocardial infarction (MI) and a 6% to 8% decrease in all-cause mortality over 10 years.[6,7] Major bleeding is the primary adverse effect of aspirin, which is most often observed in the gastrointestinal tract (rarely fatal). The risk of ICH associated with aspirin use is dose dependent. Unsurprisingly, the use of aspirin increases the potential need for surgery, morbidity, and mortality after spontaneous ICH.[8,9]

Prior to elective surgery, aspirin should be held for 7 days to 10 days prior to surgical intervention, given that aspirin provides irreversible platelet inhibition for the life span of the platelet. For patients on antiplatelet agents presenting with spontaneous or traumatic ICH, there is no reversal agent available, and some studies suggest that platelet transfusions may not improve outcomes.[10,11] Nonetheless, platelet transfusion (1 pool, $>3 \times 10^9$ platelets/L) with desmopressin (0.3 μg/kg) may be used to provide patients with uninhibited platelets (**Table 1**). Up to 5 U of platelets often are needed for sufficient clot formation, and desmopressin can be administered every 12 hours, with a maximum of 6 doses.

Although several studies have revealed no significant difference in hematoma growth or outcome after platelet transfusion,[12,13] these results are counterbalanced by numerous studies revealing a benefit. A transfusion of 10 U to 12.5 U of platelets has been shown to restore normal platelet function in patients on dual-antiplatelet regimens of aspirin and clopidogrel.[14] The administration of platelets to patients suffering from an aspirin-associated ICH has further been shown to reduce hematoma growth and mortality in several other studies as well.[15,16] The utilization of desmopressin carries some risk, particularly for patients with significant cardiac histories, but has been shown to increase platelet reactivity through the release of vWF multimers from platelet alpha-granules and Weibel-Palade bodies of endothelial cells.[17] Although the results of studies assessing the utility of these treatments remains mixed, the use of both platelet transfusion and desmopressin is recommended for severe and life-threatening ICH.

P2Y12 Inhibitors

Clopidogrel (half-life 6 hours) is a thienopyridine that irreversibly blocks the P2Y12 component of

Table 1
Reversal of antiplatelet therapeutics

Drug Class	Medication	Reversal Agent	Reversal
COX inhibitors	Aspirin	None	• Platelet transfusion (1 U pooled platelets, >3 × 10⁹/L) • Desmopressin (0.3 µg/kg, q12h)
P2Y12 inhibitors	Clopidogrel Ticagrelor Prasugrel Cangrelor	None	• Platelet transfusion (2 U pooled platelets, >3 × 10⁹/L) • Desmopressin (0.3 µg/kg, q12h)
Thromboxane inhibitors	Dipyridamole	None	• Platelet transfusion (1 U pooled platelets, >3 × 10⁹/L) • Desmopressin (0.3 µg/kg, q12h)
PDE inhibitors	Cilostazol	None	• Platelet transfusion (1 U pooled platelets, >3 × 10⁹/L) • Desmopressin (0.3 µg/kg, q12h)
Protease-activated receptor 1 inhibitors	Vorapaxar	None	• Platelet transfusion (1 U pooled platelets, >3 × 10⁹/L) • Desmopressin (0.3 µg/kg, q12h)
GP IIb/IIIa inhibitors	Abciximab Eptifibatide Tirofiban	None	• Platelet transfusion (2 U pooled platelets, >3 × 10⁹/L) • Desmopressin (0.3 µg/kg, q12h) • Cryoprecipitate

Abbreviations: PAR, protease-activated receptor; PDE, phosphodiesterase.

ADP receptors on the platelet surface, inhibiting activation of the GPIIb/IIIa receptor complex, thereby reducing platelet aggregation. Polymorphisms in the enzymes involved in the hepatic metabolism of clopidogrel to its active metabolite or within the platelet P2Y12 receptor may affect the ability of clopidogrel to inhibit platelet aggregation. Approximately one-third of patients receiving this medication are considered nonresponders and receive little to no antiplatelet benefit. This is due to a mutation in cytochrome P-450, specifically CYP-2C9 and CYP-2C19, preventing conversion of the prodrug.[18] The clinical response to the prodrug can now be adequately monitored with the VerifyNow assay (Accriva Diagnostics, San Diego, California), which measures the effect of P2Y12 inhibitors in platelet-reactive units. Clopidogrel is an oral medication, and dosing typically varies from 75 mg to 150 mg daily, after a loading dose of 300 mg to 600 mg.

Similar to clopidogrel, prasugrel (half-life 7 hours) is an oral thienopyridine prodrug, which irreversibly inhibits the P2Y12 receptor and prohibits ADP binding once converted to its active form. After a 60-mg loading dose, 10 mg per day provides effective antiplatelet function. Activation of prasugrel also requires hepatic metabolism via the same cytochrome P450 pathway (specifically CYP3A4 and CYP2B6).[19] Although prasugrel uses a similar activation pathway to clopidogrel, it does not carry the same nonresponder profile and can be successfully used in patients that may not respond to clopidogrel.

Ticagrelor (half-life 7 hours), another P2Y12 receptor inhibitor, is an orally active allosteric non-thienopyridine. After an initial loading dose of 180 mg, patients are administered 90 mg, twice daily. Unlike clopidogrel or prasugrel, ticagrelor does not require metabolic conversion to an active form, having the advantage of a more rapid and reliable onset of action. Although randomized trials have demonstrated that the use of ticagrelor, compared with clopidogrel, does decrease the risk of mortality from vascular causes, MI, or stroke, there is a significant increased risk of hemorrhage as well.[20,21] Ticagrelor is a reversible inhibitor, so platelet function normalizes after drug clearance, but there is no antidote currently available, and early data suggest that platelet transfusion has limited efficacy to reverse ticagrelor.[22]

Cangrelor (half-life 3 minutes) is a new intravenous agent that provides inhibition of the P2Y12 receptor. This fast-acting active drug does not require hepatic conversion but is quickly synthesized and cleared with platelet function returning to baseline within 1 hour of infusion.[23] Clinical use is primarily limited to patients undergoing percutaneous coronary intervention (PCI) with an active acute coronary syndrome. Given its short duration of action, transition to an oral P2Y12 inhibitor is mandatory.

In the setting of ICH or emergent surgery, the reversal of P2Y12 inhibitors is similar to that of aspirin.[24] There is no reversal agent for any of the P2Y12 inhibitors, discussed previously. Desmopressin (0.3 µg/kg) can be given every

12 hours (up to 6 doses) to induce the release of vWF and promote platelet activation and aggregation. Platelet transfusion again provides a degree of therapeutic reversal, although 2 pools (>3 × 10^9 platelets/L) of platelets are recommended, rather than 1.

Thromboxane Inhibitors

Dipyridamole (half-life 10 hours) exerts antiplatelet effects by inhibiting cAMP (cyclic adenosine monophosphate) phosphodiesterase. This in effect raises cAMP levels within platelets and reduces thromboxane A2 activity, thus interfering with platelet activation signaling pathways.[25] Despite these effects, its clinical efficacy as an antithrombotic agent is limited,[26] although the combination of aspirin and dipyridamole has been shown to be superior to aspirin alone in the prevention of secondary ischemia after an initial stroke or transient ischemic attack.[27] This drug combination is rarely used, however, due to the superiority of aspirin and P2Y12 inhibitors. Recommended dosing of dipyridamole is between 75 mg and 100 mg, dosed every 6 hours.

Reversal of the hemodynamic effects of dipyridamole can be achieved with intravenous aminophylline (or other xanthine derivatives),[28] although these agents provide little reversal of the antithrombotic effect of the drug. Similar to aspirin, platelet transfusion (1 pool, >3 × 10^9 platelets/L) and desmopressin (0.3 μg/kg) can provide sufficient substrate to facilitate coagulation and reverse the clinical effects of dipyridamole in the setting of ICH or emergent neurosurgical intervention.

Phosphodiesterase Inhibitors

Cilostazol (half-life 12 hours) is a phosphodiesterase 3 inhibitor that acts as an antiplatelet and vasodilating agent and is mainly used for intermittent claudication in patients with peripheral artery disease. Several controlled trials have found that cilostazol is effective for secondary prevention of cerebral infarction. Furthermore, cilostazol has been shown noninferior to aspirin for stroke prevention, and annual rates of hemorrhagic events (including ICH, subarachnoid hemorrhage, and other hemorrhage requiring hospitalization) are observed less frequently with cilostazol than with aspirin.[29] Similar to dipyridamole, the clinical utility of cilostazol remains minimal due to the superiority of P2Y12 inhibitors. Likewise, reversal strategies in an emergent setting mirror that of dipyridamole in which platelet transfusion (1 pool, >3 × 10^9 platelets/L) and desmopressin (0.3 μg/kg) are recommended.

Protease-activated Receptor 1 Inhibitor

Vorapaxar is an orally selective competitive antagonist of the protease-activated receptor 1, the major thrombin receptor on platelets.[30] It is currently only approved for patients with a history of MI or with peripheral artery disease. Several trials have demonstrated its efficacy in preventing thrombosis in patients undergoing PCI and in patients with atherothrombotic disease, although with a significant risk of moderate to severe bleeding, including ICH,[31] it is contraindicated in patients with previous stroke or transient ischemic attack.[32] Options for reversal are limited in the setting of ICH or emergent surgery, but treatment with platelet transfusion (1 pool, >3 × 10^9 platelets/L) and desmopressin (0.3 μg/kg) can be used.

Glycoprotein IIb/IIIa Inhibitors

As a humanized monoclonal antibody, abciximab (half-life 10–30 minutes) effectively has irreversible activity on the GP IIb/IIIa receptor due to its high affinity and slow off-rate.[33] Despite the short half-life, abciximab remains in circulation in its platelet-bound state for more than 10 days, and platelet aggregation does not resume normal function for 48 to 72 hours. Intravenous dosages typically range from 0.15 mg/kg to 0.3 mg/kg.[34] GP IIb/IIIa inhibitors were first used in patients with significant cardiac disease undergoing PCI, initially established by the EPIC trial (The Evaluation of 7E3 for the Prevention of Ischaemic Complications), which found a decrease in ischemic complications with abciximab use[35] with no significant difference in hemorrhagic stroke complications, despite an overall increase in hemorrhagic complications.[36] Since its initial use, however, several studies have found abciximab associated with an increased risk of ICH.[37,38] Nonetheless, its clinical use has continued to spread, including its use for both prophylaxis and treatment of thromboembolic complications during endovascular treatment of intracranial aneurysms.[39]

Eptifibatide (half-life 10–15 minutes) is a cyclic heptapeptide that serves as a selective, competitive GP IIb/IIIa receptor Inhibitor with a rapid onset of action.[40] Unlike abciximab, the reversal of its antiplatelet effect is much more rapid, with platelet function returning to 50% of baseline within 4 hours of infusion.

Tirofiban (half-life 2 hours) is a nonpeptide competitive inhibitor of the GP IIb/IIIa receptor as it mimics the morphology of the arginine–glycine–aspartic acid sequence of fibrinogen to prevent its binding to the receptor much like eptifibatide.[41] Given the competitive nature of its inhibition and short half-life, platelet function returns to normal within 4 hours to 8 hours of infusion.

No reversal agent exists for any of the GP IIb/IIIa receptor inhibitors, discussed previously. The primary treatment in the setting of ICH or emergent neurosurgical procedures after abciximab utilization includes platelet administration (2 pools, $>3 \times 10^9$ platelets/L), desmopressin (0.3 μg/kg every 12 hours) and drug cessation.[42] Platelet transfusion after eptifibatide or tirofiban administration is of limited use because new platelets are simply inhibited by circulating drug due to the rapid on/off pharmacokinetic properties of these small molecules. Nonetheless, in an emergent setting, platelet transfusion (2 pools, $>3 \times 10^9$ platelets/L), desmopressin (0.3 μg/kg every 12 hours)[43] and cryoprecipitate[44] have all been described.

ANTICOAGULANT THERAPEUTICS
Warfarin

Warfarin (half-life 36 hours) is the most frequently encountered oral anticoagulant, used in the treatment of venous thromboembolism (deep venous thrombosis and pulmonary embolism) and for stroke prevention in atrial fibrillation and mechanical heart valves. The mechanism of warfarin centers around vitamin K antagonism, inhibiting hepatic synthesis of vitamin K–dependent coagulation factors II, VII, IX, and X and proteins C and S, and reversal strategies are targeted at replacing these factors and the underlying synthesis of these products. Dosing warfarin can be challenging, given the influence of diet and vitamin K, but is generally initiated at 5 mg/d and is titrated to meet the international

normalized ratio (INR) goals for the necessary treatment.

Warfarin reversal strategy depends on the urgency of the associated pathology and immediacy of potential surgical intervention. If surgical intervention is not immediately imminent, particularly in cases of patients at high cardiovascular risk, discontinuation of warfarin alone may be warranted, allowing coagulation to normalize with hepatic synthesis of the inhibited coagulation factors. Oral or intravenous vitamin K may be utilized as well.

Significant, life-threatening ICH and emergent neurosurgical intervention requires immediate replacement of the inhibited coagulation factors. This may be done with either fresh frozen plasma (FFP) or prothrombin complex concentrate (PCC). PCC may be either 3-factor (factors II, IX, and X) or 4-factor (factors II, VII, IX, and X), and previous studies have shown no significant difference between the 2 forms.[15] PCC dosing largely depends on the INR of the patient at presentation (**Table 2**). Unfortunately, PCC is well known to precipitate hypercoagulability, which may lead to further venous or arterial thromboembolic complications. FFP may also be used to replace absent coagulation factors, although the need for proper blood typing delays its administration. Coupled with either FFP or PCC, vitamin K should be given as well (5–10 mg, intravenous) to facilitate autologous coagulation factor generation.[45]

Heparin

Unfractionated heparin (half-life 30–90 minutes) is classified as a factor IIa inhibitor. It binds and

Table 2
Reversal of anticoagulant therapeutics

Drug Class	Medication	Reversal Agent	Reversal

Vitamin K antagonist	Warfarin	Vitamin K	• PCC
			  ○ INR 2–4: 25 U FIX/kg
			  ○ INR 4–6: 35 U FIX/kg
			  ○ INR >6: 50 U FIX/kg
			• FFP—2 U until INR normal
			• Vitamin K—5–10 mg, intravenous

Factor IIa inhibitor	Heparin	Protamine	• Protamine 1 mg/100 U heparin over last 4 h
Factor Xa inhibitor	LMWH Fondaparinux Apixaban Rivaroxaban Edoxaban	Protamine Andexanet alfa	• Protamine 1 mg/1 mg LMWH • PCC—50 U FIX/kg • Andexanet alfa
DTIs	Bivalrudin Argatroban Dabigatran	None Praxbind	• None • Idarucizumab (Praxbind)—5 g

Abbreviations: FIX, factor IX; INR, international normalized ratio.

activates antithrombin, although it carries an unpredictable pattern of anticoagulation. At lower doses, heparin is able to inhibit factor Xa, preventing the conversion of prothrombin to thrombin; however, at higher doses it is able to inhibit numerous coagulation factors (factors IX, X, XI, and XII and thrombin) and prevent the conversion of fibrinogen to fibrin. Due to this variability, dosing ranges significantly, typically targeting a partial thromboplastin time of 2-fold above baseline,[46] although the exact range varies between institutions. Unfractionated heparin is typically used in the treatment of acute coronary syndromes, venous thromboembolic events, atrial fibrillation, open-heart surgery, and endovascular procedures.

Fortunately, protamine serves as an antidote in the setting of ICH or emergent neurosurgical procedures. Due to the overall negative charge of heparin, the positively charged protamine competes with the thrombin-binding site of heparin and effectively blocks its anticoagulation effect.[47] Dosing of protamine is dependent on the duration since the most recent heparin dose. If administered within 30 minutes, 1 mg of protamine should be given for every 100 U of heparin, whereas heparin administration 30 minutes to 120 minutes prior should be treated with 0.5 mg of protamine for every 100 U of heparin. If the most recent heparin dose was greater than 2 hours prior to reversal, 0.25 mg of protamine may be given for every 100 U of heparin, and no treatment is needed if more than 4 hours have passed. Although protamine is an effective antidote, it unfortunately dose carry significant adverse side effects of systemic hypotension and pulmonary hypertension.

Factor Xa Inhibitors

Low-molecular-weight heparins (LMWHs), half-life 3 hours to 5 hours, are administered in a subcutaneous manner and include enoxaparin, dalteparin, and tinzaparin. Initially developed to establish a more predictable course than unfractionated heparin, LMWH also binds and activates antithrombin, although with a stronger affinity to factor Xa than unfractionated heparin. Furthermore, LMWH only affects the intrinsic pathway and has no bearing on the extrinsic coagulation cascade. LMWH is typically used in venous thromboembolism prophylaxis and treatment and MI.

Although the half-life is short in duration, protamine is an adequate reversal agent in the setting of ICH or emergent surgery. Protamine dosing depends on the timing of the most recent LMWH dose. LMWH administered within 8 hours can be treated with 1 mg of protamine for every 1 mg of enoxaparin (or 100 U of dalteparin/tinazaparin), whereas a dose within 8 hours to 12 hours can be treated with 0.5 mg of protamine for every 1 mg of enoxaparin (or 100 U of dalteparin/tinazaparin). LMWH administered greater than 12 hours prior does not require protamine, because the clinical anticoagulant effect is negligible.

Fondaparinux (half-life 12–21 hours) is a heparin-related compound, serving as a selective factor Xa inhibitor, preventing the conversion of prothrombin to thrombin. It, therefore, does not inhibit thrombin directly, as observed with unfractionated heparin and LMWH.[48] Nonetheless, fondaparinux has been found similarly efficacious in terms of venous thromboembolic event and acute ischemic stroke prophylaxis,[49] with a significantly lower risk of heparin-induced thrombocytopenia despite a similar composition. It is administered subcutaneously with a daily dose of 2.5 mg.

Several orally available direct factor Xa inhibitors have been developed over the past several years. Apixaban (half-life 12 hours) is usually administered as an oral medication, 5 mg twice daily. It is most frequently used for stroke prevention in the setting of atrial fibrillation, in addition to the treatment and prevention of venous thromboembolism.[50–52] Rivaroxaban (half-life 5–9 hours) is administered as a 20-mg dose once daily and is most often used in a prophylactic manner for atrial fibrillation and for venous thromboembolic events.[53] Edoxaban (half-life 10–14 hours) is another oral anticoagulant that directly targets factor Xa. Typically administered as a once-daily 60-mg dose, it may require renal titration in patients with kidney disease.[54] It has also been shown to be efficacious in the treatment and prevention of venous thromboembolism and for stroke prevention in atrial fibrillation.[54]

In the setting of ICH and prior to emergent surgery, patients anticoagulated with fondaparinux, apixaban, rivaroxaban, and edoxaban should receive PCC (50 IU/kg) as an intravenous bolus. This has been shown to immediately and completely reverse the anticoagulant effect of factor Xa inhibitors.[55] Recently, andexanet alfa has also been approved for use in the reversal of factor Xa inhibitors, providing a robust treatment of patients suffering from an otherwise life-threatening hemorrhage. Andexanet is a recombinant modified human factor Xa decoy protein that is able to bind factor Xa inhibitors with high affinity.[56]

Recent studies have shown that andexanet alfa provides complete reversal of these inhibitors within minutes of administration.[56,57] Andexanet dosing is time sensitive. Patients receiving a factor Xa inhibitor within 7 hours should be treated with 800-mg bolus, followed by a 960-mg infusion over 2 hours. If the most recent dose is greater than 7 hours prior to andexanet administration, a 400-mg bolus, followed by a 480-mg infusion over 2 hours should be given.[56]

Direct Thrombin Inhibitors

Bivalirudin (half-life 25 minutes) is an intravenously administered DTI, binding to both the active site and exosite I of thrombin. It provides reversible inhibition of thrombin-mediated platelet activation and aggregation. Bivalirudin is typically used in the treatment of unstable angina, MI, PCI, stroke prevention in the setting of atrial fibrillation, and venous thromboembolic treatment and for heparin-induced thrombocytopenia.[58]

A reversible inhibitor, aragtroban (half-life 40 minutes) similarly binds directly to the active site of thrombin but not to exosite I. It is typically administered in an intravenous manner in the prevention of atrial fibrillation-associated stroke, venous thromboembolism prevention, and the management of heparin-induced thrombocytopenia.[59] Typically dosed between 2 μg/kg to 10 μg/kg per minute, its therapeutic efficacy is achieved when the partial thromboplastin time is 1.5-fold to 3-fold above baseline levels.

Finally, dabigatran (half-life 8 hours) is another DTI, administered as an oral medication, with a dose of 150 mg twice daily.[60] It is primarily used in the prophylaxis and treatment of venous thromboembolism, stroke prevention in atrial fibrillation, and heparin-induced thrombocytopenia.

Bivalirudin and argatroban have no antidotes or other agents that can reliably reverse their anticoagulant properties. In severe life-threatening emergencies, 50 IU/kg PCC may be attempted.[45] Fortunately, an antibody fragment (idarucizumab) was developed to reverse the anticoagulant effects of dabigatran.[61] In the setting of ICH or emergent surgery, idarucizumab [5 g], may be intravenously administered, because this has been shown to completely reverse the effect of dabigatran within minutes.

SUMMARY

Although antiplatelet and anticoagulation therapeutics can have drastic consequences in patients suffering from ICH or in need of an emergent neurosurgical procedure, numerous strategies exist to ameliorate their effect and restore normal hemostasis. Fortunately, in drug classes previously without appropriate reversal strategies, newer antidotes have shown promise in limiting catastrophic hemorrhage. As newer agents continue to be developed, it will be imperative for the practicing neurosurgeon to continue to remain up to date on reversal strategies given the potential significant side effects of these drug classes.

REFERENCES

1. Sarode R, Matevosyan K, Bhagat R, et al. Rapid warfarin reversal: a 3-factor prothrombin complex concentrate and recombinant factor VIIa cocktail for intracerebral hemorrhage. J Neurosurg 2012; 116(3):491–7.
2. Balami JS, Buchan AM. Complications of intracerebral haemorrhage. Lancet Neurol 2012;11(1): 101–18.
3. Wintzen AR, de Jonge H, Loeliger EA, et al. The risk of intracerebral hemorrhage during oral anticoagulant treatment: a population study. Ann Neurol 1984;16(5):553–8.
4. Hoffman M. Remodeling the blood coagulation cascade. J Thromb Thrombolysis 2003;16(1–2): 17–20.
5. Hoffman M, Monroe DM 3rd. A cell-based model of hemostasis. Thromb Haemost 2001;85(6):958–65.
6. Rothwell PM, Price JF, Fowkes FG, et al. Short-term effects of daily aspirin on cancer incidence, mortality, and non-vascular death: analysis of the time course of risks and benefits in 51 randomised controlled trials. Lancet 2012;379(9826):1602–12.
7. Guirguis-Blake JM, Evans CV, Senger CA, et al. Aspirin for the primary prevention of cardiovascular events: a systematic evidence review for the U.S. preventive services task force. Ann Intern Med 2016;164(12):804–13.
8. Naidech AM, Bernstein RA, Levasseur K, et al. Platelet activity and outcome after intracerebral hemorrhage. Ann Neurol 2009;65(3):352–6.
9. Naidech AM, Jovanovic B, Liebling S, et al. Reduced platelet activity is associated with early clot growth and worse 3-month outcome after intracerebral hemorrhage. Stroke 2009;40(7):2398–401.
10. Martin M, Conlon LW. Does platelet transfusion improve outcomes in patients with spontaneous or traumatic intracerebral hemorrhage? Ann Emerg Med 2013;61(1):58–61.
11. Baharoglu MI, Cordonnier C, Al-Shahi Salman R, et al. Platelet transfusion versus standard care after acute stroke due to spontaneous cerebral haemorrhage associated with antiplatelet therapy (PATCH): a randomised, open-label, phase 3 trial. Lancet 2016;387(10038):2605–13.
12. Ducruet AF, Hickman ZL, Zacharia BE, et al. Impact of platelet transfusion on hematoma expansion in patients receiving antiplatelet agents before intracerebral hemorrhage. Neurol Res 2010;32(7):706–10.
13. Nishijima DK, Zehtabchi S, Berrong J, et al. Utility of platelet transfusion in adult patients with traumatic intracranial hemorrhage and preinjury antiplatelet

use: a systematic review. J Trauma Acute Care Surg 2012;72(6):1658–63.

14. Vilahur G, Choi BG, Zafar MU, et al. Normalization of platelet reactivity in clopidogrel-treated subjects. J Thromb Haemost 2007;5(1):82–90.

15. Beshay JE, Morgan H, Madden C, et al. Emergency reversal of anticoagulation and antiplatelet therapies in neurosurgical patients. J Neurosurg 2010;112(2): 307–18.

16. McMillian WD, Rogers FB. Management of prehospital antiplatelet and anticoagulant therapy in traumatic head injury: a review. J Trauma 2009;66(3): 942–50.

17. Flordal PA, Sahlin S. Use of desmopressin to prevent bleeding complications in patients treated with aspirin. Br J Surg 1993;80(6):723–4.

18. Patrono C, Baigent C, Hirsh J, et al. Antiplatelet drugs: American college of chest physicians evidence-based clinical practice guidelines (8th edition). Chest 2008;133(6 Suppl):199S–233S.

19. Schror K, Siller-Matula JM, Huber K. Pharmacokinetic basis of the antiplatelet action of prasugrel. Fundam Clin Pharmacol 2012;26(1):39–46.

20. Wallentin L, Becker RC, Budaj A, et al. Ticagrelor versus clopidogrel in patients with acute coronary syndromes. N Engl J Med 2009;361(11):1045–57.

21. DiNicolantonio JJ, D'Ascenzo F, Tomek A, et al. Clopidogrel is safer than ticagrelor in regard to bleeds: a closer look at the PLATO trial. Int J Cardiol 2013; 168(3):1739–44.

22. Godier A, Taylor G, Gaussem P. Inefficacy of platelet transfusion to reverse ticagrelor. N Engl J Med 2015; 372(2):196–7.

23. Qamar A, Bhatt DL. Current status of data on cangrelor. Pharmacol Ther 2016;159:102–9.

24. Sarode R. How do I transfuse platelets (PLTs) to reverse anti-PLT drug effect? Transfusion 2012; 52(4):695–701 [quiz: 694].

25. Schwarz UR, Walter U, Eigenthaler M. Taming platelets with cyclic nucleotides. Biochem Pharmacol 2001;62(9):1153–61.

26. Diener HC, Cunha L, Forbes C, et al. European Stroke Prevention Study. 2. Dipyridamole and acetylsalicylic acid in the secondary prevention of stroke. J Neurol Sci 1996;143(1–2):1–13.

27. Halkes PH, Gray LJ, Bath PM, et al. Dipyridamole plus aspirin versus aspirin alone in secondary prevention after TIA or stroke: a meta-analysis by risk. J Neurol Neurosurg Psychiatry 2008;79(11): 1218–23.

28. Johnson NP, Lance Gould K. Dipyridamole reversal using theophylline during aminophylline shortage. J Nucl Cardiol 2011;18(6):1115.

29. Shinohara Y, Katayama Y, Uchiyama S, et al. Cilostazol for prevention of secondary stroke (CSPS 2): an aspirin-controlled, double-blind, randomised non-inferiority trial. Lancet Neurol 2010;9(10):959–68.

30. Magnani G, Bonaca MP, Braunwald E, et al. Efficacy and safety of vorapaxar as approved for clinical use in the United States. J Am Heart Assoc 2015;4(3): e001505.

31. Morrow DA, Braunwald E, Bonaca MP, et al. Vorapaxar in the secondary prevention of atherothrombotic events. N Engl J Med 2012;366(15):1404–13.

32. Tricoci P, Huang Z, Held C, et al. Thrombin-receptor antagonist vorapaxar in acute coronary syndromes. N Engl J Med 2012;366(1):20–33.

33. Fiorella D, Albuquerque FC, Han P, et al. Strategies for the management of intraprocedural thromboembolic complications with abciximab (ReoPro). Neurosurgery 2004;54(5):1089–97 [discussion: 1097–8].

34. Altenburg A, Haage P. Antiplatelet and anticoagulant drugs in interventional radiology. Cardiovasc Intervent Radiol 2012;35(1):30–42.

35. Investigators E. Use of a monoclonal antibody directed against the platelet glycoprotein IIb/IIIa receptor in high-risk coronary angioplasty. N Engl J Med 1994;330(14):956–61.

36. Califf RM, Lincoff AM, Tcheng JE, et al. An overview of the results of the EPIC trial. Eur Heart J 1995; 16(Suppl L):43–9.

37. Walsh RD, Barrett KM, Aguilar MI, et al. Intracranial hemorrhage following neuroendovascular procedures with abciximab is associated with high mortality: a multicenter series. Neurocrit Care 2011;15(1): 85–95.

38. Cho YD, Lee JY, Seo JH, et al. Early recurrent hemorrhage after coil embolization in ruptured intracranial aneurysms. Neuroradiology 2012;54(7):719–26.

39. Dornbos D 3rd, Katz JS, Youssef P, et al. Glycoprotein IIb/IIIa inhibitors in prevention and rescue treatment of thromboembolic complications during endovascular embolization of intracranial aneurysms. Neurosurgery 2018;82(3):268–77.

40. Sedat J, Chau Y, Gaudard J, et al. Administration of eptifibatide during endovascular treatment of ruptured cerebral aneurysms reduces the rate of thromboembolic events. Neuroradiology 2015; 57(2):197–203.

41. Sedat J, Chau Y, Mondot L, et al. Is eptifibatide a safe and effective rescue therapy in thromboembolic events complicating cerebral aneurysm coil embolization? Single-center experience in 42 cases and review of the literature. Neuroradiology 2014; 56(2):145–53.

42. Tcheng JE. Clinical challenges of platelet glycoprotein IIb/IIIa receptor inhibitor therapy: bleeding, reversal, thrombocytopenia, and retreatment. Am Heart J 2000;139(2 Pt 2):S38–45.

43. Reiter RA, Mayr F, Blazicek H, et al. Desmopressin antagonizes the in vitro platelet dysfunction induced by GPIIb/IIIa inhibitors and aspirin. Blood 2003; 102(13):4594–9.

44. Li YF, Spencer FA, Becker RC. Comparative efficacy of fibrinogen and platelet supplementation on the in vitro reversibility of competitive glycoprotein IIb/IIIa (alphaIIb/beta3) receptor-directed platelet inhibition. Am Heart J 2001;142(2):204–10.

45. van Ryn J, Stangier J, Haertter S, et al. Dabigatran etexilate–a novel, reversible, oral direct thrombin inhibitor: interpretation of coagulation assays and reversal of anticoagulant activity. Thromb Haemost 2010;103(6):1116–27.

46. Hirsh J, Warkentin TE, Shaughnessy SG, et al. Heparin and low-molecular-weight heparin: mechanisms of action, pharmacokinetics, dosing, monitoring, efficacy, and safety. Chest 2001;119(1 Suppl):64S–94S.

47. Hirsh J, Anand SS, Halperin JL, et al, American Heart Association. Guide to anticoagulant therapy: Heparin: a statement for healthcare professionals from the American Heart Association. Circulation 2001;103(24):2994–3018.

48. Bijsterveld NR, Moons AH, Boekholdt SM, et al. Ability of recombinant factor VIIa to reverse the anticoagulant effect of the pentasaccharide fondaparinux in healthy volunteers. Circulation 2002;106(20):2550–4.

49. Hackett CT, Ramanathan RS, Malhotra K, et al. Safety of venous thromboembolism prophylaxis with fondaparinux in ischemic stroke. Thromb Res 2015;135(2):249–54.

50. Potpara TS, Polovina MM, Licina MM, et al. Novel oral anticoagulants for stroke prevention in atrial fibrillation: focus on apixaban. Adv Ther 2012;29(6):491–507.

51. Granger CB, Alexander JH, McMurray JJ, et al. Apixaban versus warfarin in patients with atrial fibrillation. N Engl J Med 2011;365(11):981–92.

52. O'Donnell MJ, Eikelboom JW, Yusuf S, et al. Effect of apixaban on brain infarction and microbleeds: AVERROES-MRI assessment study. Am Heart J 2016;178:145–50.

53. Perzborn E, Roehrig S, Straub A, et al. Rivaroxaban: a new oral factor Xa inhibitor. Arterioscler Thromb Vasc Biol 2010;30(3):376–81.

54. Poulakos M, Walker JN, Baig U, et al. Edoxaban: a direct oral anticoagulant. Am J Health Syst Pharm 2017;74(3):117–29.

55. Eerenberg ES, Kamphuisen PW, Sijpkens MK, et al. Reversal of rivaroxaban and dabigatran by prothrombin complex concentrate: a randomized, placebo-controlled, crossover study in healthy subjects. Circulation 2011;124(14):1573–9.

56. Connolly SJ, Milling TJ Jr, Eikelboom JW, et al. Andexanet alfa for acute major bleeding associated with factor Xa inhibitors. N Engl J Med 2016;375(12):1131–41.

57. Siegal DM, Curnutte JT, Connolly SJ, et al. Andexanet alfa for the reversal of factor Xa inhibitor activity. N Engl J Med 2015;373(25):2413–24.

58. Stone GW, McLaurin BT, Cox DA, et al. Bivalirudin for patients with acute coronary syndromes. N Engl J Med 2006;355(21):2203–16.

59. Lewis BE, Wallis DE, Leya F, et al. Argatroban anticoagulation in patients with heparin-induced thrombocytopenia. Arch Intern Med 2003;163(15):1849–56.

60. Connolly SJ, Ezekowitz MD, Yusuf S, et al. Dabigatran versus warfarin in patients with atrial fibrillation. N Engl J Med 2009;361(12):1139–51.

61. Pollack CV Jr, Reilly PA, Eikelboom J, et al. Idarucizumab for dabigatran reversal. N Engl J Med 2015;373(6):511–20.

Section III: Coagulation in the Perioperative Patient

Intraoperative Blood and Coagulation Factor Replacement During Neurosurgery

James J. Zhou, MD, Tsinsue Chen, MD, Peter Nakaji, MD*

KEYWORDS

- Blood components • Blood replacement • Blood transfusion • Coagulation
- Intraoperative procedures

KEY POINTS

- The decision to transfuse during a neurosurgical procedure should be based on multiple data points, including vital signs, laboratory studies, and observations of the surgical field.
- Up-to-date knowledge on available blood products, components, and factors is critical when deciding when and how to replete a neurosurgery patient intraoperatively.
- The type of neurosurgical procedure, underlying pathologic condition, and surgical technique all influence the probability of requiring an intraoperative transfusion.

INTRODUCTION

In the late nineteenth century, the field of neurosurgery struggled with perioperative mortality rates of 30% to 50%. Of the many drivers of perioperative mortality, one of the most significant was large-volume intraoperative blood loss. Any significant blood loss during surgery presented a major challenge because of a lack of understanding regarding blood types and compatibility, an inability to store blood for extended periods of time, and a paucity of available donors intraoperatively.[1]

The safe transfusion of blood products to counteract intraoperative bleeding became possible in the twentieth century after several advances. In 1901, Karl Landsteiner published his seminal work on the 4 primary blood groups, but his findings were not widely adopted until the 1920s. ABO terminology was not accepted until the 1937 Congress of the International Society of Blood Transfusion. In 1943, based on the work of Richard Lewinsohn, Peyton Rous, and J. R. Turner, the use of citrate-phosphate-dextrose solution was adopted, allowing for the anticoagulation and storage of blood for up to 28 days before transfusion—a development that led to blood banks. Finally, 2 landmark contributions by Edwin Cohn (the fractionation of plasma proteins with ethyl alcohol in 1946 and the first cell separator developed in 1951) paved the way for modern-day blood component therapy.[2]

In this article, the authors review the use of intraoperative blood and coagulation factor replacement as it pertains to modern neurosurgical practice. Various methods of assessing hemodynamic and coagulation status intraoperatively are discussed, as are blood components and coagulation factors available for transfusion. Updated

Disclosures: The authors have nothing to disclose.
Department of Neurosurgery, Barrow Neurological Institute, St. Joseph's Hospital and Medical Center, 350 West Thomas Road, Phoenix, AZ 85013, USA
* Corresponding author. Neuroscience Publications, Barrow Neurological Institute, St. Joseph's Hospital and Medical Center, 350 West Thomas Road, Phoenix, AZ 85013.
E-mail address: Neuropub@barrowneuro.org

Neurosurg Clin N Am 29 (2018) 547–555
https://doi.org/10.1016/j.nec.2018.06.006
1042-3680/18/© 2018 Elsevier Inc. All rights reserved.

information is provided on current strategies for intraoperative transfusion in cranial and spinal surgery and on the management of patients whose personal beliefs preclude transfusion.

INTRAOPERATIVE ASSESSMENT OF HEMODYNAMIC AND COAGULATION STATUS

Many of the same techniques used during the preoperative workup can also be used to evaluate hemodynamic and coagulation status during neurosurgery. Because many patients begin surgery with both intravenous and arterial access, it is not difficult to repeat any routine hematologic laboratory studies, platelet function assays, or even thromboelastography several times during a procedure.

Determining when it is appropriate to reassess hemodynamic and coagulation status intraoperatively begins with clinical observations, including the degree of blood loss from the surgical field and the presence or absence of normal clot formation with routine hemostatic maneuvers (eg, electrocautery, topical hemostatic agents). The patient's vital signs should also be observed closely. Physiologic indicators of blood loss (eg, reduced urine output, tachycardia, narrowed pulse pressure, hypotension, hypoxemia) may signal the need for earlier laboratory evaluation. Intraoperative assessments (eg, complete blood count, prothrombin time [PT], international normalized ratio [INR], activated partial thromboplastin time [aPTT]) can be compared with the patient's preoperative baseline when considering transfusion.

Other common laboratory studies not routinely conducted preoperatively may provide valuable insight on a patient's coagulation state during surgery. Fibrinogen, fibrin degradation product, and D-dimer levels provide useful information about ongoing processes related to coagulation. Fibrinogen is the terminal target of the coagulation cascade and is continuously consumed during surgery as fibrin clots form. A fibrinogen level of greater than 100 to 200 mg/dL is typically sufficient to provide normal clotting function; however, lower levels may prompt repletion with cryoprecipitate or a different fibrinogen-containing transfusate.[3] Furthermore, serial measurements of plasma fibrinogen may help detect consumptive coagulopathy, such as disseminated intravascular coagulation (DIC). Fibrin degradation product and D-dimer levels from fibrinolysis may also indicate ongoing DIC if abnormally elevated.

Thromboelastography is increasingly popular for monitoring coagulation status intraoperatively. Thromboelastography-guided transfusion algorithms have been shown to reduce perioperative

fresh frozen plasma (FFP) transfusion requirements in multiple surgical specialties (eg, hepatic surgery, cardiac surgery, neurosurgery).[4–6] Intraoperative thromboelastography can also be used to identify patients at high risk for excessive bleeding, and in some cases, thromboelastography has proved superior to more conventional measures such as platelet count.[7,8] Furthermore, neurosurgical reports indicate that hypocoagulability measured on perioperative thromboelastography may predict increased risk of postoperative hematoma in pediatric patients undergoing craniotomy for primary brain tumors.[9]

Other novel modalities for monitoring hematologic and coagulation parameters have also been explored. For example, pulse CO-oximetry has been demonstrated to provide a noninvasive, relatively accurate estimate of hemoglobin concentration using a fingertip sensor. Continuous, noninvasive hemoglobin monitoring also reduces the need for intraoperative blood transfusions during elective orthopedic surgery.[10] A recent systematic review demonstrated good overall correlation between mean CO-oximetry measurements and traditional laboratory measurements, but noted a wide range of agreement ($\pm$2.2–3.0 perioperatively), which may limit the utility of CO-oximetry for guiding clinical decision making.[11] Point-of-care hemoglobinometers have also been demonstrated to correlate closely with traditional laboratory hematology analyzers intraoperatively and may provide another rapid, nominally invasive means of hemoglobin monitoring.[12]

The importance of monitoring hematologic and coagulation status intraoperatively is best illustrated by DIC, which is a potentially catastrophic hematologic complication of surgery, particularly cranial neurosurgery. DIC is a consumptive coagulopathy characterized by widespread, systemic activation of primary and secondary coagulation. This activation can cause extensive thrombus formation in the microvasculature of multiple organ systems, resulting in dysfunction. During surgery, ongoing activation of the coagulation cascade consumes plasma anticoagulants such as antithrombin III, protein C, and tissue factor (TF) inhibitor, thus predisposing patients to overactivation of the coagulation cascade. The systemic release of TF during cranial neurosurgery because of manipulation of brain tissue may further contribute to hyperactivation of the TF pathway of secondary hemostasis.

The clinical phenotype of DIC during surgery varies, depending on the balance between plasma thrombin and plasmin levels, and it may range from extensive thrombosis to abnormal, persistent bleeding from the surgical field. No single laboratory test can diagnose DIC, which reinforces the importance of continuously monitoring the status of ongoing coagulation using the previously described methods. Closely observing and interpreting trends in routine laboratory studies (eg, PT, aPTT, platelet count, fibrinogen, fibrin degradation products, D-dimer) is critical to identifying DIC. Thromboelastography for global assessment of hemostasis can provide further insight into the balance between coagulation and fibrinolysis during DIC and may help guide treatment.

INTRAOPERATIVE BLOOD AND COAGULATION FACTOR REPLACEMENT

During surgical procedures, it often becomes necessary to transfuse blood products to maintain tissue oxygenation, promote hemostasis, and counteract consumptive coagulopathy. Various blood-derived transfusates, including individual blood components and isolated coagulation factors, can be administered to counteract the natural loss or consumption of these elements during surgery. Moreover, numerous nonblood substances, such as desmopressin (DDAVP; Ferring Pharmaceuticals, Inc, Parsippany, NJ, USA), antifibrinolytics, and protease inhibitors, can also be given to promote or inhibit the function of blood components. Neurosurgeons should therefore become familiar with all options available to address intraoperative hematologic disturbances.

Available Blood Components and Coagulation Factors

Packed red blood cells

The administration of packed red blood cells (pRBC) during surgery helps preserve the oxygen-carrying capacity of blood when there is rapid or significant blood loss. One unit of pRBC has an intrinsic hematocrit of 0.55 to 0.80 and a total volume of 225 to 250 mL. Assuming a closed system, one unit should increase hemoglobin by 1 g/dL and hematocrit by 0.03 for an average-sized adult patient.

Randomized cardiac surgery trials have demonstrated that restrictive perioperative hemoglobin transfusion thresholds, defined variably as less than 7.5 to 8.0 g/dL, produce outcomes similar to those for more liberal transfusion thresholds regarding 30-day mortality, ischemic events, and infection.[13–15] These studies have also found that restrictive transfusion thresholds reduce the number of patients exposed to transfusions, thus reducing the risk of transfusion-related adverse events. However, there have been no randomized controlled neurosurgery trials to guide transfusion

thresholds in patients undergoing cranial or spinal surgery.

Although restrictive transfusion strategies may be appropriate for most patients and procedures, evidence suggests that more liberal transfusion thresholds may be better in certain patient populations. For example, the CRIT trial of anemia and blood transfusion in critically ill patients demonstrated that a nadir hemoglobin level of less than 9 g/dL was an independent predictor for increased mortality and length of hospitalization.[16] Other cardiac surgery research has shown that an intraoperative hemoglobin decrease greater than 50% from preoperative baseline was associated with worse outcomes, even if absolute hemoglobin remained greater than 7 g/dL.[17] Thus, the decision to transfuse pRBC during neurosurgery is multifactorial and should consider all relevant data, including type of surgery, patient demographics and medical and surgical history, blood pressure, oxygen saturation, preoperative and intraoperative hemoglobin levels, and the amount and rate of observed blood loss. Supplemental tests (eg, point-of care hemoglobin, pulse CO-oximetry) may also further define intraoperative trends in hemoglobin levels.

When deciding whether to transfuse pRBC, one must also consider the potential for negative results. In addition to the well-documented risks of acute hemolysis and infection transmission associated with allogeneic transfusions, intraoperative administration of pRBC may increase the likelihood of pneumonia, sepsis, ischemic outcomes, and 30-day morbidity and mortality.[18] Intraoperative pRBC transfusions may even increase 1-year mortality in a dose-dependent manner.[19]

Platelets

Platelets are transfused during surgery to prevent or halt bleeding related to thrombocytopenia or platelet dysfunction. In the operating room, platelets are essential to normal primary hemostasis and to the function of topical hemostatic agents (eg, microfibrillar collagens; microporous polysaccharide hemospheres—artificial matrices that require an intact primary hemostatic pathway). Platelets are transfused as pheresis-collected single-donor units containing approximately 3 to 6×10^{11} platelets per pack. Although the response may vary if the administered platelets are immediately consumed or sequestered, transfusion with one single-donor unit should increase the total platelet count by about 50,000 platelets per microliter.

Intraoperative platelet transfusion goals are largely derived from expert recommendations and retrospective studies. A minimum platelet count of 100,000 platelets per microliter should be maintained throughout an operation and for at least 48 to 72 hours afterward. Intraoperative platelet transfusion may also aid hemostasis in nonthrombocytopenic patients with known platelet dysfunction, such as patients on aspirin or clopidogrel therapy. Similar to pRBC transfusion, platelet transfusion may increase 1-year mortality in a dose-dependent manner.[20] Other potential complications include anaphylaxis, febrile nonhemolytic transfusion reactions, and disease transmission.

Fresh frozen plasma

Fresh frozen plasma (FFP) is transfused intraoperatively to correct coagulation factor deficiencies. These factors are necessary not only for the normal formation of fibrin clots in response to surgical trauma but also for the proper functioning of any non-thrombin-soaked topical hemostatic agent. Coagulation factor deficiencies may occur for multiple reasons, including blood loss, hemophilia, warfarin therapy, or DIC. In addition, FFP is administered to patients who require massive infusions of pRBC, platelets, or crystalloids or colloids to avoid excessive dilution of endogenous clotting factors. One FFP unit is approximately 200 to 250 mL; each unit contains 1 unit/mL of each coagulation factor and 2 mg/mL of fibrinogen. FFP has an intrinsic INR of 0.9 to 1.2; thus, infusion of FFP can only be expected to correct a patient's INR to 1.2 to 1.3. Because the half-life of the most hemostatically relevant factor (factor VII) is approximately 5 hours, FFP must be administered continuously until a more durable treatment, such as vitamin K replacement, has taken effect.

The decision to give FFP during surgery may be based on several variables. For example, abnormal or up-trending PT, INR, and aPTT values may signal the need to replete coagulation factors with FFP, especially after abnormal bleeding. One common practice is to transfuse FFP to maintain PT, INR, and aPTT values at less than 1.5 times the control values for abnormal bleeding. Intraoperative thromboelastography can also be used to guide FFP infusions. Studies of patients undergoing orthotopic liver transplantation and complex cardiac surgery have shown that thromboelastography-guided transfusion algorithms can reduce FFP transfusion requirements without affecting overall outcomes.[4,5] The typical threshold for FFP transfusion is abnormal bleeding coupled with an R value greater than 2 times the control on intraoperative thromboelastography.

Prothrombin complex concentrate

Prothrombin complex concentrate (PCC) consists of precipitated concentrates of various coagulation factors produced by ion-exchange chromatography on the cryoprecipitate of large donated plasma pools. Either 3-factor PCC (containing factors II, IX, and X) or 4-factor PCC (containing factors II, VII, IX, and X) is produced, depending on the type of ion-exchange chromatography. Different PCCs are available from different manufacturers, each containing different proportions of coagulation factors. Some 4-factor PCCs, such as the factor IX complex Bebulin VH (Baxter AG, Vienna, Austria), contain minimal factor VII. Others, such as Prothromplex T (Baxter AG), contain near-equal amounts of all 4 factors. In neurosurgery, PCC has historically been used for rapid correction of warfarin therapy, especially in patients with intracranial hemorrhage.[21,22] However, PCC is also used to correct coagulation factor deficiencies from various causes, including liver failure, massive transfusion, and hemophilia B, and other congenital coagulation factor deficiencies.[23,24]

During neurosurgery, both PCC and FFP are used for similar indications, but PCC offers several advantages. First, PCC does not require thawing or compatibility testing before use, allowing for more rapid administration. Second, PCC also contains a much larger concentration of coagulation factors per unit volume, which allows for more rapid and complete correction of PT and INR without risk of volume overload.[25,26] Finally, the manufacturing of PCC involves a viral reduction process, which reduces the risk of infectious disease transmission.[26]

Despite these advantages, PCC has been associated with a high incidence of thrombotic complications, including deep vein thrombosis, pulmonary embolus, myocardial infarction, and cerebrovascular accident. Although the source of this thrombogenicity is uncertain, it may relate to the high concentration of factor II in PCC. The risk of thrombotic complications is increased by liver disease, antithrombin III deficiency, and large, repetitive doses of PCC. The potential for these adverse effects must be weighed when considering intraoperative PCC administration.[26,27]

Cryoprecipitate

Cryoprecipitate is created by centrifuging FFP and collecting the precipitate. The resulting preparation contains fibrinogen, von Willebrand factor, factor VIII, and factor XIII (fibrin-stabilizing factor). In clinical practice, cryoprecipitate may be administered to correct conditions causing deficiencies in any of these factors, including hemophilia, von Willebrand disease, massive transfusion, and DIC. Notably, adequate fibrinogen levels are necessary for the formation of normal fibrin clots as well as for the proper functioning of any thrombin-soaked topical hemostatic agent. A fibrinogen level of 100 mg/dL may be sufficient for normal hemostasis, but in vitro data support 200 mg/dL for optimal clot formation.[28]

In neurosurgery, cryoprecipitate is most often administered to correct low fibrinogen levels that typically occur due to consumption of fibrinogen caused by ongoing clotting or dilution of intrinsic fibrinogen levels caused by transfusion of other blood products. Hypofibrinogenemia may be the most common dilutional coagulopathy observed during neurosurgery, albeit perhaps underappreciated because fibrinogen levels are not routinely monitored.[29] The conventional trigger for fibrinogen replacement is 100 mg/dL, although the threshold may be raised to 200 mg/dL because of the heightened risk of hemorrhagic morbidity and mortality in neurosurgery patients.[29–31]

Individual coagulation factor concentrates

Several individual coagulation factor concentrates can assist with targeted factor repletion and hemostasis in neurosurgery patients: factors I, VII, VIII, and IX. Of these, recombinant factor VIIa (rFVIIa; NovoSeven; Novo Nordisk, A/S, Bagsvaerd, Denmark) has undergone extensive study in neurosurgery patients and is frequently used for numerous indications.

rFVIIa acts locally on TF-containing cells at sites of tissue injury and vascular wall disruption. It promotes hemostasis by forming a complex with TF, resulting in thrombin production and platelet activation. It also directly converts factor X to Xa on the surface of activated platelets, initiating a "thrombin burst" that accelerates the coagulation cascade at the injury site. Although rFVIIa was approved by the US Food and Drug Administration only for use in patients with hemophilia who have antibodies to factor VIII or IX, it is often used off-label to reverse anticoagulation, to prevent intracranial hemorrhage progression, and to reduce surgical bleeding. It has been shown to be highly effective in correcting abnormalities in PT and INR. Almost all series demonstrate that rFVIIa administration rapidly corrects INR values to the reference range, even in patients with severe coagulopathies and INR greater than 10.[32,33] INR correction with rFVIIa has also been shown to occur more quickly than with FFP alone.[34]

Although no official recommendations exist for the intraoperative use of rFVIIa in neurosurgery patients, it is reportedly useful for prophylaxis or treatment of severe intraoperative bleeding.[35–37] However, existing supportive data are from low-quality, nonrandomized trials. Further study is necessary to determine whether intraoperative rFVIIa is more effective than more traditional agents.

Tranexamic acid

Tranexamic acid (TXA) is a synthetic lysine analogue that acts as a competitive inhibitor of intrinsic plasmin and plasminogen. It saturates the lysine-binding sites of plasminogen, displacing it from fibrin surfaces and preventing fibrinolysis. This action accelerates the relative rate of fibrin clot formation as compared with fibrinolysis, theoretically allowing for more rapid hemostasis and reduced blood loss. Although not traditionally used in routine intraoperative blood and coagulation factor replacement, TXA has been increasingly used during neurosurgery to prevent excessive blood loss and reduce transfusion requirements.

When TXA is preoperatively loaded and continuously administered intraoperatively, it has been shown to reduce blood loss and transfusions. Multiple randomized, controlled trials have demonstrated that TXA reduces intraoperative and postoperative blood loss and transfusions in several neurosurgery subspecialties, including pediatric scoliosis surgery, pediatric craniosynostosis surgery, and routine and complex adult spine surgery.[38–41] Nonrandomized data in other neurosurgery disciplines, including complex skull base surgery, have also demonstrated its efficacy in reducing intraoperative blood loss and transfusions.[42] One meta-analysis also showed that TXA was effective in reducing operating times in spine surgery.[43] Accepted doses of TXA vary widely. Pediatric neurosurgery patients have used loading doses ranging from 10 to 30 mg/kg, followed by continuous infusions of up to $\leq$1 mg/kg/h.[38] Adult neurosurgery patients, especially complex spine patients, typically receive higher overall doses, with a loading dose of 10 to 25 mg/kg followed by continuous infusions of 5 to 10 mg/kg/h.[39]

Despite support for the use of TXA during neurosurgery, its use is not without complications. Studies of cardiac surgery patients have shown that TXA is associated with increased risk of seizures, persistent atrial fibrillation, and renal failure.[44] However, most randomized, controlled trials in the neurosurgery literature have not found an association between TXA and increased thromboembolic complications.[38,42] Overall, specific recommendations regarding when to use TXA in neurosurgery patients have yet to be formulated. The decision should be based on careful consideration of numerous variables, including type of surgery, expected blood loss, and conditions increasing thromboembolic risk.

Intraoperative Transfusion in Cranial Neurosurgery

Although many cranial neurosurgery procedures can be completed with minimal blood loss, any unanticipated intraoperative or postoperative bleeding may have serious consequences. Because of the high metabolic and oxygen requirements of brain tissue, hypoxia secondary to blood loss anemia or mass effect can cause widespread tissue ischemia and neuronal death, especially after traumatic brain injury or surgery. Studies of patients with traumatic brain injury have shown that hemoglobin less than 9 g/dL and brain tissue oxygen tension less than 20 mm Hg are independently associated with poor outcomes.[45,46] Intracranial mass effect may also cause cerebral herniation, resulting in devastating, irreversible neurologic deficits and death. Therefore, maintenance of proper blood and coagulation parameters during cranial neurosurgery is critical.

Determining when to transfuse a patient undergoing cranial neurosurgery begins with preoperative planning. The type of procedure influences the probability that a blood or coagulation factor transfusion will be required. Reported pRBC transfusion rates range from 10% for complex, skull-based tumors to 45% for pediatric synostosis.[42,47,48] Surgical technique and underlying pathologic condition may also help predict the need for a blood transfusion. Some research indicates that patients undergoing aneurysm clipping have an average pRBC transfusion rate of 25%; however, the risk of transfusion increases dramatically with higher preoperative risk scores or an intraoperative rupture.[49] Finally, preoperative laboratory evaluations are crucial in identifying patients more likely to require an intraoperative transfusion, such as patients with anemia or preexisting coagulopathies.

Given the potential complications of unplanned or uncontrollable intracranial bleeding during cranial neurosurgery, neurosurgeons should maintain a low threshold for intraoperative transfusion during these procedures. Monitoring blood and coagulation parameters should complement continuous monitoring of the surgical field to allow the surgeon to formulate a complete picture of the patient's coagulation status. Deficiencies in any factor required for hemostasis (eg, platelets, individual coagulation factors) should be promptly corrected to preempt abnormal bleeding. If bleeding does not adequately respond to routine blood and coagulation factor resuscitation, rFVIIa or TXA may be administered. Finally, although significant blood loss anemia is rare in most cranial neurosurgery cases, hemoglobin and hematocrit levels should be monitored, and appropriate transfusion should be performed when necessary to maintain adequate brain tissue oxygenation.

Intraoperative Transfusion in Spinal Neurosurgery

Similar to brain tissue, spinal cord tissue is exquisitely sensitive to both hypoxia and mass effect. Therefore, many of the transfusion principles for cranial neurosurgery also apply to spinal procedures. However, unlike cranial cases, spinal cases frequently involve extensive disruption of soft tissue and bone, creating an opportunity for significant blood loss.

Preoperative planning is therefore critical to estimating the need for intraoperative transfusion. Patients with normal hematologic parameters who are undergoing relatively minor spine surgery (eg, elective cervical or lumbar procedures) are less likely to need transfusions of pRBC or coagulation factors to correct for intraoperative blood loss. The average rate of pRBC transfusion in elective cervical fusion procedures is approximately 1.47%, with patients undergoing multilevel procedures more likely to require transfusion.[50] The estimated rate of pRBC transfusion in elective lumbar fusions is also relatively low (about 6%), with longer operating times and lower preoperative hemoglobin predictive of transfusion requirements.[51] Because these patients have low anticipated transfusion requirements, surgeons may elect to proceed without placing blood or coagulation factors on hold, as long as careful hemostasis is maintained. Conversely, patients undergoing large spinal procedures, such as adult spinal deformity correction, are much more likely to require intraoperative transfusion. In one large series, 46.5% of patients undergoing such correction required intraoperative or postoperative blood transfusion.[52] In patients with high anticipated blood loss, blood components should be on standby to preempt the development of anemia and coagulopathy due to intraoperative blood loss. Systemic hemostatic agents such as rFVIIa and TXA can also be considered if excessive blood loss is anticipated or if unmanageable bleeding is encountered. As with all neurosurgery cases, meticulous hemostasis and continuous evaluation of the patient's hematologic status are essential.

Coagulation Factor and Component Replacement in Jehovah's Witnesses

Patients who will not accept blood product transfusion, such as Jehovah's Witnesses, require individualized management with regard to intraoperative blood and coagulation factor transfusion. Most Jehovah's Witnesses will not accept transfusion of whole blood or any fractionated blood components (eg, pRBC, platelets, plasma) based on interpretations of biblical passages stating that blood cannot be consumed as nourishment. On an individual basis, some persons who identify as Jehovah's Witnesses may accept cryoprecipitate, plasma proteins (eg, albumin, immunoglobulin), isolated coagulation factors, and autologous blood preserved in a Cell Saver (Haemonetics Corp, Braintree, MA, USA). Given these limitations, correcting for blood loss or coagulopathies is highly challenging in these patients. However, hemodynamic and coagulation status can be optimized preoperatively using nutritional supplements such as iron, vitamin B12, and folate. Intraoperatively, efforts should be made to minimize blood loss to avoid acute anemia or coagulopathy. In cases of acute anemia, erythropoiesis-stimulating agents may restore hemoglobin. However, these agents are not true replacements for transfusion, given new RBC production requires several weeks.[53] Overall, management of patients such as Jehovah's Witnesses must be carefully individualized based on patient preferences and on preoperative and intraoperative hemodynamic status.

SUMMARY

Intraoperative blood and coagulation factor replacement in neurosurgery cases is a complex and multifactorial issue that requires frequent and careful assessment of the patient's hemodynamic and coagulation status. The enormous heterogeneity that exists among neurosurgery patients precludes comprehensive recommendations regarding blood and coagulation factor replacement that apply to all patients in all situations. Rather, each patient should be evaluated individually, and adequate blood and coagulation factor replacement should be initiated based on informed and reasoned clinical judgment.

ACKNOWLEDGMENTS

The authors thank the staff of Neuroscience Publications at Barrow Neurological Institute for assistance with article preparation.

REFERENCES

1. Voorhees JR, Cohen-Gadol AA, Spencer DD. Early evolution of neurological surgery: conquering increased intracranial pressure, infection, and blood loss. Neurosurg Focus 2005;18(4):e2.
2. Giangrande PL. The history of blood transfusion. Br J Haematol 2000;110(4):758–67.
3. Loftus CM. Anticoagulation and hemostasis in neurosurgery. New York: Springer Science+Business Media; 2016.
4. Shore-Lesserson L, Manspeizer HE, DePerio M, et al. Thromboelastography-guided transfusion algorithm reduces transfusions in complex cardiac surgery. Anesth Analg 1999;88(2):312–9.
5. Wang SC, Shieh JF, Chang KY, et al. Thromboelastography-guided transfusion decreases intraoperative blood transfusion during orthotopic liver transplantation: randomized clinical trial. Transplant Proc 2010;42(7):2590–3.
6. Israelian LA, Gromova VV, Lubnin A. Reducing the frequency of fresh frozen donor plasma transfusion on the basis of the results of thromboelastographic study in neurosurgical patients with intraoperative blood loss. Anesteziol Reanimatol 2009;(5):28–32 [in Russian].
7. Essell JH, Martin TJ, Salinas J, et al. Comparison of thromboelastography to bleeding time and standard coagulation tests in patients after cardiopulmonary bypass. J Cardiothorac Vasc Anesth 1993;7(4):410–5.
8. Williams GD, Bratton SL, Riley EC, et al. Coagulation tests during cardiopulmonary bypass correlate with blood loss in children undergoing cardiac surgery. J Cardiothorac Vasc Anesth 1999;13(4):398–404.
9. El Kady N, Khedr H, Yosry M, et al. Perioperative assessment of coagulation in paediatric neurosurgical patients using thromboelastography. Eur J Anaesthesiol 2009;26(4):293–7.
10. Ehrenfeld JM, Henneman JP, Sandberg W. Impact of continuous and noninvasive hemoglobin monitoring on intraoperative blood transfusions. Paper presented at: Proceedings of the Annual Meeting of the American Society Anesthesiologists, San Diego, CA, USA, October 16–20, 2010.
11. Kim SH, Lilot M, Murphy LS, et al. Accuracy of continuous noninvasive hemoglobin monitoring: a systematic review and meta-analysis. Anesth Analg 2014;119(2):332–46.
12. Giraud B, Frasca D, Debaene B, et al. Comparison of haemoglobin measurement methods in the operating theatre. Br J Anaesth 2013;111(6):946–54.
13. Mazer CD, Whitlock RP, Fergusson DA, et al. Restrictive or liberal red-cell transfusion for cardiac surgery. N Engl J Med 2017;377(22):2133–44.
14. Hajjar LA, Vincent JL, Galas FR, et al. Transfusion requirements after cardiac surgery: the TRACS

randomized controlled trial. JAMA 2010;304(14): 1559–67.

15. Bracey AW, Radovancevic R, Riggs SA, et al. Lowering the hemoglobin threshold for transfusion in coronary artery bypass procedures: effect on patient outcome. Transfusion 1999;39(10):1070–7.

16. Corwin HL, Gettinger A, Pearl RG, et al. The CRIT study: anemia and blood transfusion in the critically ill – current clinical practice in the United States. Crit Care Med 2004;32(1):39–52.

17. Hogervorst E, Rosseel P, van der Bom J, et al. Tolerance of intraoperative hemoglobin decrease during cardiac surgery. Transfusion 2014;54(10 Pt 2):2696–704.

18. Bernard AC, Davenport DL, Chang PK, et al. Intraoperative transfusion of 1 U to 2 U packed red blood cells is associated with increased 30-day mortality, surgical-site infection, pneumonia, and sepsis in general surgery patients. J Am Coll Surg 2009; 208(5):931–7, 937.e1–2; [discussion: 938–939].

19. Murphy GJ, Reeves BC, Rogers CA, et al. Increased mortality, postoperative morbidity, and cost after red blood cell transfusion in patients having cardiac surgery. Circulation 2007;116(22):2544–52.

20. de Boer MT, Christensen MC, Asmussen M, et al. The impact of intraoperative transfusion of platelets and red blood cells on survival after liver transplantation. Anesth Analg 2008;106(1):32–44.

21. Cartmill M, Dolan G, Byrne JL, et al. Prothrombin complex concentrate for oral anticoagulant reversal in neurosurgical emergencies. Br J Neurosurg 2000;14(5):458–61.

22. Boulis NM, Bobek MP, Schmaier A, et al. Use of factor IX complex in warfarin-related intracranial hemorrhage. Neurosurgery 1999;45(5):1113–9.

23. Siddon AJ, Tormey CA. Successful use of four factor-prothrombin complex concentrate for congenital factor X deficiency in the setting of neurosurgery. Lab Med 2016;47(3):e35–7.

24. Gerlach R, Krause M, Seifert V, et al. Hemostatic and hemorrhagic problems in neurosurgical patients. Acta Neurochir (Wien) 2009;151(8):873–900.

25. Goldstein JN, Refaai MA, Milling TJ Jr, et al. Four-factor prothrombin complex concentrate versus plasma for rapid vitamin K antagonist reversal in patients needing urgent surgical or invasive interventions: a phase 3b, open-label, non-inferiority, randomised trial. Lancet 2015;385(9982):2077–87.

26. Sorensen B, Spahn DR, Innerhofer P, et al. Clinical review: prothrombin complex concentrates–evaluation of safety and thrombogenicity. Crit Care 2011;15(1):201.

27. Kohler M. Thrombogenicity of prothrombin complex concentrates. Thromb Res 1999;95(4 Suppl 1):S13–7.

28. Bolliger D, Szlam F, Molinaro RJ, et al. Finding the optimal concentration range for fibrinogen replacement after severe haemodilution: an in vitro model. Br J Anaesth 2009;102(6):793–9.

29. Nair S, Nair BR, Vidyasagar A, et al. Importance of fibrinogen in dilutional coagulopathy after neurosurgical procedures: a descriptive study. Indian J Anaesth 2016;60(8):542–5.

30. Practice parameter for the use of fresh-frozen plasma, cryoprecipitate, and platelets. Fresh-Frozen Plasma, Cryoprecipitate, and Platelets Administration Practice Guidelines Development Task Force of the College of American Pathologists. JAMA 1994;271(10):777–81.

31. Spahn DR, Bouillon B, Cerny V, et al. Management of bleeding and coagulopathy following major trauma: an updated European guideline. Crit Care 2013; 17(2):R76.

32. Mayer SA, Brun NC, Begtrup K, et al. Efficacy and safety of recombinant activated factor VII for acute intracerebral hemorrhage. N Engl J Med 2008; 358(20):2127–37.

33. Deveras RA, Kessler CM. Reversal of warfarin-induced excessive anticoagulation with recombinant human factor VIIa concentrate. Ann Intern Med 2002;137(11):884–8.

34. Brody DL, Aiyagari V, Shackleford AM, et al. Use of recombinant factor VIIa in patients with warfarin-associated intracranial hemorrhage. Neurocrit Care 2005;2(3):263–7.

35. Kapapa T, König K, Heissler HE, et al. The use of recombinant activated factor VII in neurosurgery. World Neurosurg 2009;71(2):172–9.

36. Heisel M, Nagib M, Madsen L, et al. Use of recombinant factor VIIa (rFVIIa) to control intraoperative bleeding in pediatric brain tumor patients. Pediatr Blood Cancer 2004;43(6):703–5.

37. Vesel AS, Novak-Jankovič V, Maldini B, et al. Use of recombinant activated factor VIIa in a-six-month-old child due to massive hemorrhage during elective surgery for choroid plexus carcinoma: case report. Acta Clin Croat 2015;54(3):381–7.

38. Neilipovitz DT, Murto K, Hall L, et al. A randomized trial of tranexamic acid to reduce blood transfusion for scoliosis surgery. Anesth Analg 2001;93(1):82–7.

39. Elwatidy S, Jamjoom Z, Elgamal E, et al. Efficacy and safety of prophylactic large dose of tranexamic acid in spine surgery: a prospective, randomized, double-blind, placebo-controlled study. Spine (Phila Pa 1976) 2008;33(24):2577–80.

40. Alajmi T, Saeed H, Alfaryan K, et al. Efficacy of tranexamic acid in reducing blood loss and blood transfusion in idiopathic scoliosis: a systematic review and meta-analysis. J Spine Surg 2017;3(4): 531–40.

41. Goobie SM, Meier PM, Pereira LM, et al. Efficacy of tranexamic acid in pediatric craniosynostosis surgery: a double-blind, placebo-controlled trial. Anesthesiology 2011;114(4):862–71.

42. Mebel D, Akagami R, Flexman AM. Use of tranexamic acid is associated with reduced blood product

transfusion in complex skull base neurosurgical procedures: a retrospective cohort study. Anesth Analg 2016;122(2):503–8.

43. Hui S, Xu D, Ren Z, et al. Can tranexamic acid conserve blood and save operative time in spinal surgeries? A meta-analysis. Spine J 2017. [Epub ahead of print].

44. Martin K, Wiesner G, Breuer T, et al. The risks of aprotinin and tranexamic acid in cardiac surgery: a one-year follow-up of 1188 consecutive patients. Anesth Analg 2008;107(6):1783–90.

45. Griesdale DE, Sekhon MS, Menon DK, et al. Hemoglobin area and time index above 90 g/L are associated with improved 6-month functional outcomes in patients with severe traumatic brain injury. Neurocrit Care 2015;23(1):78–84.

46. Oddo M, Levine JM, Kumar M, et al. Anemia and brain oxygen after severe traumatic brain injury. Intensive Care Med 2012;38(9):1497–504.

47. Dadure C, Sauter M, Bringuier S, et al. Intraoperative tranexamic acid reduces blood transfusion in children undergoing craniosynostosis surgery: a randomized double-blind study. Anesthesiology 2011; 114(4):856–61.

48. White N, Marcus R, Dover S, et al. Predictors of blood loss in fronto-orbital advancement and remodeling. J Craniofac Surg 2009;20(2):378–81.

49. Luostarinen T, Lehto H, Skrifvars MB, et al. Transfusion frequency of red blood cells, fresh frozen plasma, and platelets during ruptured cerebral aneurysm surgery. World Neurosurg 2015;84(2): 446–50.

50. Aoude A, Aldebeyan S, Fortin M, et al. Prevalence and complications of postoperative transfusion for cervical fusion procedures in spine surgery: an analysis of 11,588 patients from the American College of Surgeons National Surgical Quality Improvement Program database. Asian Spine J 2017;11(6):880–91.

51. Ristagno G, Beluffi S, Tanzi D, et al. Red blood cell transfusion need for elective primary posterior lumbar fusion in a high-volume center for spine surgery. J Clin Med 2018;7(2):19–30.

52. Durand WM, DePasse JM, Daniels AH. Predictive modeling for blood transfusion following adult spinal deformity surgery: a tree-based machine learning approach. Spine (Phila Pa 1976) 2017. [Epub ahead of print].

53. Mann MC, Votto J, Kambe J, et al. Management of the severely anemic patient who refuses transfusion: lessons learned during the care of a Jehovah's witness. Ann Intern Med 1992;117(12): 1042–8.

Management of Intraoperative Coagulopathy

Michal Bar-Natan, MD, Kenneth B. Hymes, MD*

KEYWORDS

- Coagulopathy • Anticoagulant • Disseminated intravascular coagulation (DIC)
- Prothrombin complex concentrates (PCC) • Tranexamic acid/antifibrinolytics
- Recombinant factor VIIa (rFVIIa)

KEY POINTS

- Intraoperative hemorrhage can occur even in optimally prepared patients let alone during urgent procedures. Identifying the reason is crucial for appropriate and timely fashioned treatment.
- The cornerstone treatment of disseminated intravascular coagulation is transfusion therapy to correct the consumption of platelets and coagulation factors.
- Urgent reversal treatment of vitamin K antagonists–associated life-threatening bleeding includes vitamin K and prothrombin complex concentrate.
- Using recombinant factor VIIa should be considered for intractable bleeding when all other therapies have failed to achieve hemostasis.
- Antifibrinolytic therapy, such as tranexamic acid, should be considered as prophylaxis treatment before major surgery and to treat bleeding due to fibrinolysis.

Achieving and maintaining hemostasis during neurosurgical procedures is critical to their successful outcomes. Although the risk of hemorrhage can often be predicted with preoperative laboratory screening and a complete history and physical examination, there remain patients in whom intraoperative hemorrhage cannot be predicted.

The coagulation system is a complex interplay between cellular and molecular components. Hemostasis is a dynamic process that needs to be rapid, localized, and highly regulated. There is a balance between thrombus formation and lysis, and surgical trauma may disrupt this balance and cause abnormal bleeding or excessive thrombosis.

There is a difference between an elective procedure when preparation is optimal (good history, preoperative evaluation, and interruption of anticoagulant medications) versus urgent/emergent surgery when patients are often receiving antiplatelet agents, vitamin K antagonists (VKAs), or a direct oral anticoagulant (DOAC). In addition, in an emergency, no information about medications, concomitant medical conditions, or bleeding history may be available. Thus, the lack of reliable clinical information may contribute to unanticipated intraoperative hemorrhage.

Patients can bleed because of the surgical procedure or because of an impaired ability to establish hemostasis. In this review, the authors do not discuss technical factors that lead to intraoperative hemorrhage. The authors review potential causes for disrupted hemostasis, including a brief overview of the preparation for urgent procedures in patients on anticoagulants and the therapeutic options.

Disclosure Statement: The authors have nothing to disclose.

Division of Hematology and Oncology, Department of Internal Medicine, Laura and Isaac Perlmutter Cancer Center, New York University School of Medicine, 240 East 38th Street, 19th Floor, New York, NY 10016, USA

* Corresponding author.

E-mail address: Kenneth.Hymes@nyumc.org

Neurosurg Clin N Am 29 (2018) 557–565

https://doi.org/10.1016/j.nec.2018.06.007

It is extremely important to identify either acquired or inherited hemostatic defects if bleeding is encountered. The history should be reevaluated (if possible). In addition, the preoperative medications, including crystalloids, colloids, and blood products, should be reassessed. The laboratory evaluation that will screen for coagulation defects, including thrombocytopenia (or platelet dysfunction), should be reviewed in the context of intraoperative hemorrhage. It is also important to collect several tubes of citrated plasma before the administration of a blood product or other hemostatic agents in order to obtain a baseline assessment of hemostatic function.

Pharmacologic treatments for excessive bleeding include

- Topical hemostatics (eg, fibrin glue, thrombin gel)
- Transfusion of platelets
- Transfusion of coagulation factor concentrates: fresh frozen plasma (FFP), prothrombin complex concentrate (PCC), and recombinant factor VIIa (rFVIIa)
- Antifibrinolytics (ε-aminocaproic acid, tranexamic acid [TXA])
- Treatments for hypofibrinogenemia (cryoprecipitate, fibrinogen concentrate)
- Desmopressin (DDAVP).

INTRAOPERATIVE DISSEMINATED INTRAVASCULAR COAGULATION/ COAGULOPATHY

Disseminated intravascular coagulation (DIC) is a clinicopathologic condition in which there is intravascular activation of the coagulation system and regulators. This activation leads to the generation of soluble fibrin monomers, which deposit in the microvasculature and cause organ damage. There is simultaneous platelet and coagulation factor consumption and depletion, which may lead to bleeding. The pathophysiology of DIC is complex. It is well known that traumatic brain injury (TBI) is associated with severe coagulopathy, and existence of such at presentation is a predictor of unfavorable outcomes.[1] Multiple mechanisms are potentially linked to coagulopathy after TBI including disorders of platelet number and function, changes in endogenous procoagulant and anticoagulant factors, endothelial cell activation, hypoperfusion, and inflammation.

The causes of these hemostatic changes are not completely understood but likely include the release of tissue factor (TF) from the damaged brain, which binds extensively to factor VIIa triggering the extrinsic coagulation pathway, which results in thrombin generation. Platelets are activated by several mechanisms, first by local tissue or vessel injury (eg, exposed subendothelial matrix) and second by cytokine and TF release by systemically activated endothelial cells (eg, related to shock), possible platelet hyperactivity with subsequent platelet consumption, and secondary platelet depletion and dysfunction. Overactivation of clotting via TF has been suggested to drive hyperfibrinolysis. In addition, brain injury can promote clot dissolution by release of tissue-type and urokinase-type plasminogen activators. As multiple thrombi form, the systemic consumption of fibrinogen and platelets leads to bleeding complications.[1]

Even though very uncommon, there are case reports of DIC developing during neurosurgical removal of a tumor; this is associated with a high mortality rate.[2–4] It is thought to be related in part to tumor TF expression, a major actor in the activation of the coagulation cascade.

DIAGNOSIS

The diagnosis of DIC includes a combination of clinical and laboratory parameters. No single test can verify or exclude the diagnosis. It is also a dynamic situation that may necessitate serial clinical and laboratory evaluation.

An analysis of 5 reports of patient groups with DIC, with a total of more than 900 patients, suggests that the laboratory abnormalities reported in decreasing the order of frequency are thrombocytopenia, elevated fibrin degradation products, prolonged prothrombin time (PT), prolonged activated partial thromboplastin time (PTT), and low fibrinogen.[5]

The International Society of Thrombosis and Hemostasis recommended the use of a scoring system for overt DIC, whereby the presence of an underlying disorder known to be associated with DIC was a prerequisite for the use of the algorithm. It consists of simple tests (platelet number, PT, D-dimer, fibrin degradation products, and fibrinogen [**Table 1**]). It was found to be both sensitive (91%) and specific (97%) for the diagnosis of DIC, and an increased score correlated with an increase in the odds of mortality.[6,7]

Although the literature about the use of this scoring system during surgery is lacking, trauma was one of the specified prerequisites for an underlying disorder associated with DIC.

Other methods to identify coagulopathy during surgery include using viscoelastic hemostatic assays (VHAs), such as thromboelastography (TEG) or rotational thromboelastometry (ROTEM). These assays are point-of-care assays, capable of global assessments of coagulation based on the physical and kinetic properties of clot formation, that

Table 1
International Society of Thrombosis and Hemostasis's disseminated intravascular coagulation scoring system

Parameter	Results	Score
Platelet count	>100 × 10⁹/L	0
	50 × 10⁹/L – 100 × 10⁹/L	1
	<50 × 10⁹/L	2
PT prolongation	3 s or less	0
	>3 s but <6 s	1
	>6 s	2
Fibrin markers (D-dimer, FDP)	No change	0
	Moderate increase (<10 times normal)	2
	Strong increase	3
Fibrinogen	>1 g/L	0
	<1 g/L	1

Five or greater compatible with overt DIC: repeat score daily.
   Less than 5 suggestive for nonovert DIC: repeat next 1 to 2 days.
   Abbreviation: FDP, fibrin degradation products.

account for the cellular and plasma components of coagulation. These tests are performed on whole blood and allow for a quick evaluation of all phases of hemostasis (initiation, propagation, strength, and dissolution). They are thought to represent a more physiologic evaluation (eg, reflect the cell-based model of hemostasis, clotting factor, and platelet interactions) of the coagulation system.[8]

The use of VHAs might be of higher importance in patients treated with DOAC (especially when they need urgent neurosurgical intervention) when the conventional coagulation tests are less capable of assessing their effect. Furthermore, VHAs can be valuable in treating patients with TBI with unknown prior exposure to anticoagulant or antiplatelet drugs, whereby they might predict the risk of traumatic hematoma expansion and the need for urgent surgical intervention.

There are case reports of successful use of these techniques in neurosurgery (eg, treatment with TXA when results were suggestive of fibrinolysis)[2,9]; however, randomized clinical data are sparse. A recent comprehensive review and meta-analysis of the use of TEG and ROTEM in bleeding patients, which included 1493 patients in 17 trials (mostly of elective cardiac surgery, excision of burn wounds and liver transplantation), shows that using this technique seems to reduce the overall mortality and incidence of transfusion; but the quality of evidence is low.[10] Moreover, a Cochrane review of VHAs in trauma does not show that TEG/ROTEM could definitively diagnose early traumatic coagulopathy.[11]

In a recent prospective observational study comparing standard coagulation tests (SCTs) with VHA, in 92 patients undergoing emergent neurosurgery a coagulopathic pattern was detected preoperatively in 35% patients based on SCTs and in 21% based on ROTEM analysis. The results obtained with ROTEM correlated with SCTs. ROTEM assays were equal or superior to SCTs in identifying patients with acute coagulopathy and in predicting intraoperative blood transfusion requirement. Moreover, the administration of platelet concentrates, PCC, FFP, fibrinogen, and TXA could be guided using well-established thresholds. The investigators concluded that ROTEM was an effective tool and could provide valuable information regarding the causes of perioperative hemorrhage especially because of its rapid turn-around time.[12]

The European Society of Anesthesiology recommends the use of VHAs for monitoring perioperative hemostasis in neurosurgery, but the recommendation is only graded 2C (weak recommendation with low-quality evidence).[13]

TREATMENT

The cornerstone of treating DIC is treating the underlying cause. Of course in cases of trauma this is not always possible.

The principal treatment of bleeding patients with DIC is transfusion therapy.

TRANSFUSION

The British guidelines[5] suggest platelet transfusions to a different threshold according to the clinical situation. Transfusion for platelet counts of less than 100,000/μL in bleeding neurosurgical patients is a reasonable value, but it has not been studied in a randomized controlled trial.

Patients with prolonged PT/PTT with bleeding or a high risk for bleeding should be transfused with FFP (initial doses of 15 mL/kg); if patients are fluid overloaded, consider using factor concentrates, such as PCC. Of note, FFP given at volumes of greater than 15 mg/kg are less effective because of the dilution of the coagulation factors.

Importantly, there are no specific PT/PTT/international normalized ratio (INR) values to be achieved, and the correlation between a mildly elevated INR and hemorrhage is imperfect[14]; therefore, clinical judgment should be used.

Severe hypofibrinogenemia (<1 g/L) may be treated with cryoprecipitate in order to obtain a concentration threshold of 1.5 to 2.0 g/L.[15]

In general, patients with DIC should not be treated with antifibrinolytic agents. There are rare patients with DIC in whom hyperfibrinolysis predominates over intravascular thrombosis. In these patients, severe bleeding could be treated with antifibrinolytic agents, such as TXA (see later discussion); but there is a risk of developing thromboses.

PROTHROMBIN COMPLEX CONCENTRATES

PCCs are plasma-derived products. Three different types are available: 3 factor PCCs contain factors II, IX, and X along with small amounts of factor VII. Four factor PCCs contain factors II, IX, and X and also therapeutically adequate amounts of factor VII. Activated PCCs contains 4 factors, including activated factor VII. Four factor PCCs are most effective in rapid INR correction in VKA-induced anticoagulation, as they replace all vitamin K–dependent factors.[13,16]

Data for PCCs use for urgent reversal of anticoagulation in acutely bleeding patients (intracranial hemorrhage [ICH], trauma, or before urgent surgery) come from retrospective case reports/series as well as prospective clinical trials. It is well established that PCCs can rapidly and effectively reduce INR and achieve adequate hemostasis in patients treated with VKA.[17–23]

In a recent systematic review, 21 studies with a total of 4783 VKA-treated patients were included. Reversal treatment was given for ICH (n = 2202), other major bleeding (n = 1642), before urgent invasive intervention (n = 596), or other reasons (n = 320). Treatment with 4 factor PCCs led to an INR of 1.5 or less in 63.0% of patients (as compared with 12.2% in patients treated with FFP). Thromboembolic events were reported in 1.63% of PCC-treated patients. Clinical benefit assessment was not possible.[24]

For urgent reversal of VKA and for severe perioperative bleeding in patients on VKA, administration of PCCs is recommended by both the American and European (grade 1B recommendation) societies of anesthesiology.[15,25]

Data for PCC use for reversal of DOAC are less abundant. In the UPRATE (Unactivated Prothrombin Complex Concentrates for the Reversal of Anti-factor Ten Inhibitors) prospective study, 84 patients received 4-factor PCCs (25 IU/kg median dose 2000 IU) for the urgent reversal of the anticoagulant effect of rivaroxaban or apixaban due to a major bleeding events (70% ICH, 15% gastrointestinal bleeding). The treatment was hemostatically effective in 69.1% of the patients. Two cases of ischemic stroke and one case of suspected pulmonary embolism were observed. The 30-day mortality was 32%.[26] In a recently published German multicenter observational analysis of 146 patients

with DOAC-related ICH (131 patients with factor Xa inhibitor [rivaroxaban, apixaban], 15 with dabigatran), hematoma enlargement occurred in 33.6%. There were no significant differences between those with PCC treatment (median dose 2000 IU) compared with those without regarding the rate of hematoma enlargement, mortality, or functional outcome at 3 months.[27]

The guidelines for reversal of antithrombotics in ICH recommend administering a 4-factor PCC (50 U/kg) or activated PCC (50 U/kg) if ICH is associated with direct anti-Xa drug exposure.[28] Of note, idarucizumab is approved by the US Food and Drug Administration (FDA) for the reversal of dabigatran in life-threatening or uncontrolled bleeding based on the RE-VERSE AD trial (Reversal effects of Idarucizumab on active dabigatran).[29] In addition, the FDA has also approved andexanet for the similar indications.[30]

There are few published data on the use of PCCs in bleeding related to surgery. A retrospective report of 24 patients (cardiac surgery [7], other surgery [9], warfarin [Warfarin] reversal [8]) with a poor response to transfusion of FFP, platelets, and cryoprecipitate (defined as continued bleeding despite near correction of clotting parameters) who received PCCs showed that partial or complete hemostasis was achieved in 77.8%.[31] Another retro review reported on 41 acute care surgery patients (mostly trauma or emergency surgery) with coagulopathy who received a low dose (15 IU/kg) of PCC. Of the 12 patients who were not taking prehospital Warfarin, 75% had a successful correction of INR; one event of venous thromboembolism was observed in the whole cohort.[32]

In patients with excessive bleeding and increased INR not related to VKA use, who are not responding to other component transfusion, use of PCCs is a reasonable therapy.

RECOMBINANT FACTOR VIIa

The mechanism of action of rFVIIa is via its binding to the surface of activated platelets, increasing activation of FIX and FX, and increasing thrombin generation to greater than normal levels.[33]

This product is currently US FDA approved for treating or preventing bleeding in hemophilic patients who have antibody inhibitors to coagulation factors VIII or IX, treating or preventing bleeding in patients with acquired hemophilia, and patients with congenital factor VII deficiency. It is also licensed in Europe for the treatment of Glanzmann thrombasthenia.

The half-life of rFVIIa in the circulation is 2 hours; certain conditions, such as hypothermia, acidosis, electrolyte disturbances, and loss of coagulation factors and/or platelets secondary to consumption or dilution by fluid administration, can impact its effectiveness.[34]

rFVIIa has been used in a wide range of clinical scenarios when patients have intractable bleeding and all other therapies have failed to achieve hemostasis. There are numerous case reports and some clinical trials of its use in bleeding patients on a wide variety use of anticoagulants, trauma, platelet dysfunction, and liver failure, including case reports of successful off-labeled use of rFVIIa in massive bleeding during neurosurgical surgery.[35,36]

In a phase 3 trial, 841 patients with spontaneous ICH (not associated with anticoagulant use) received hemostatic therapy with rFVIIa or placebo within 4 hours after the onset of symptoms. The rFVIIa treatment reduced the growth of the hematoma but did not improve survival or functional outcome at 3 months.[37] A later systematic review of the use of rFVIIa for 5 off-label indications was published. The meta-analysis for ICH included 4 randomized controlled trials including more than 900 patients, none of whom were on anticoagulation. Use of rFVIIa significantly decreased relative hematoma expansion at all doses. It did not have an effect on overall survival or functional outcome compared with the standard of care. However, there was an increased rate of arterial thromboembolism in the medium-high-dose group.[38]

For patients on anticoagulants and ICH, for Warfarin users the treatment usually includes vitamin K, FFP (large volume), or PCCs. The routine use of rFVIIa is usually not recommended. A retrospective review of 101 patients with Warfarin-associated ICH (54% had ICH and 30% subdural hematomas) of whom 42.5% had neurosurgical intervention, who received rFVIIa (mean dose 51.7 mcg/kg), rFVIIa (in conjunction with other treatments) rapidly reversed INR; but thromboembolic complications were reported in 8 patients.[39]

In another retrospective review, 58 patients presenting with ICH (41% subdural), of whom 43 were on Warfarin and 1 on dabigatran, 84% were taken to surgery. INR was rapidly corrected in this cohort with an average rFVIIa dose of 73 mcg/kg, and only 3% had thromboembolic complications.[40]

There are no data comparing outcomes in this group of patients. Of note, normalizing INR may not reflect full reversal of coagulopathy because the INR is particularly sensitive to factor VII levels. INR correction may occur despite inadequate levels of other factors (II, IX, X) that are required for hemostasis. Moreover, because of rFVIIa's short half-life, this normalization could be of short duration. Currently, rFVIIa is not recommended for reversal of VKA in ICH.[28]

For bleeding patients on DOAC, although clinical data are lacking, results from preclinical/in vitro studies seem to be conflicting, with some data indicating that rFVIIa is less effective than other hemostatic agents (ie, activated or nonactivated PCCs).[41–43]

Antifibrinolytics ε-Aminocaproic Acid, Tranexamic Acid

The mechanism of action is as follows: TXA reversibly blocks lysine-binding sites on plasminogen molecules, thereby preventing its conversion to plasmin and inhibiting fibrin clot dissolution.

The use of antifibrinolytics has been investigated for decades. The largest earlier randomized controlled trial included 479 patients with subarachnoid hemorrhage (SAH) who were treated with TXA versus placebo within 72 hours and up to 28 days. The rate of rebleeding was reduced from 24% to 9%, but concurrently there was an increase in ischemic complications (24% vs 15%). This finding translated to no difference in outcome at 3 months.[44] Later a prospective trial of 504 patients showed that the administration of 1.0 g of TXA immediately after the diagnosis of aneurysmal SAH followed by 1.0 g every 6 hours until aneurysmal occlusion (no more than 72 hours) reduced the early rebleeding from 10.8% to 2.4% and showed an 80% reduction in the mortality rate from early rebleeding with no increased risk of either ischemic clinical manifestations or vasospasm attributed to TXA.[45] A Cochrane review of antifibrinolytic treatment of aneurismal SAH showed a reduction in the risk of rebleeding (relative risk [RR] 0.64); but the RR for reported cerebral ischemia was 1.41, and death and outcome were similar.[46] An ongoing phase 3 large international trial, the Tranexamic Acid for Hyperacute Primary Intra Cerebral Hemorrhage (TICH-2) trial, is designed to determine if TXA can improve outcomes in spontaneous intracerebral hemorrhage (ISRCTN93732214).

The efficacy and safety for the use of antifibrinolytic in intracranial surgery are not well established.

Early results showed that intraoperative administration of aprotinin reduced blood lost in meningioma/vestibular schwannoma surgeries in patients not receiving anticoagulation.[47] However, subsequent results in cardiac surgery showed that aprotinin was associated with a modest reduction of massive bleeding but also with a significantly higher risk of death[48]; it was removed from the market by the US FDA.

A retrospective analysis reported 519 patients undergoing skull base neurosurgical procedures in a single institution, of whom 245 received TXA (average total dose 37 mg/kg).

The rate of perioperative transfusion in patients who received TXA was significantly lower (7% vs 13%, $P = .04$), and the rates of seizure and thromboembolic events were similar between the two groups.[49] Additionally, another retrospective analysis of 119 patients undergoing cervical laminectomy with lateral mass screw fixation and bone grafting reported 73 patients who received TXA (15 mg/kg before skin incision followed by 100 mg/h until skin closure). Intraoperative and postoperative blood loss was significantly lower in the TXA group relative to the control group with no major intraoperative or postoperative complications, including a thromboembolic complication, observed in either group.[50]

A recent systematic review of the literature showed that systemic IV TXA is an efficacious hemostatic agent in spinal surgery, reducing perioperative blood loss and blood transfusion requirements. Use of topical TXA in surgery suggests similar hemostatic efficacy with potentially improved safety as compared with intravenous TXA.[51]

The European Society of Anesthesiology recommends using TXA to prevent bleeding during major surgery and/or treat bleeding due to (at least suspected) fibrinolysis (dose 20–25 mg/kg) (grade 1B recommendation).[15] The American Society of Anesthesiology recommends using prophylactic antifibrinolytic therapy in patients undergoing cardiopulmonary bypass and considering prophylactic antifibrinolytic therapy to reduce bleeding and the risk of transfusion for patients at risk of excessive bleeding.[25]

As stated previously, TBI is associated with coagulopathy. Increased fibrinolysis could be a part of this coagulopathy and can increase the bleeding. The Clinical Randomization of an Antifibrinolytic in Significant Hemorrhage (CRASH-2) trial was conducted in 20,211 bleeding trauma patients. The Intracranial Bleeding Study (CRASH-2 IBS) was conducted nested within the CRASH-2 trial. Two hundred seventy patients were randomized to receive a loading dose of 1.0 g of TXA infused over 10 minutes, followed by an intravenous infusion of 1.0 g over 8 hours (133 patients) or matching placebo. The results showed a nonsignificant reduction in hematoma growth. All-cause mortality was 10.5% in the TXA group versus 17.5% in the placebo group (adjusted odds ratio [OR] for death was 0.49 [95% CI 0.22–1.06]). Forty-five percent of patients in the TXA group and 58% in the placebo group had a poor outcome (adjusted OR for poor outcome was 0.57 [95% CI 0.33–0.98]).[52] Another trial randomized 238 patients with TBI to receive

either TXA (single dose of 2.0 g) or placebo. They found that progression of ICH in the TXA-treated group was lower than in the placebo group (27% vs 18%, RR 0.65, 95% confidence interval 0.40–1.05). No differences in death or unfavorable outcomes were observed between treatment groups, and there was no increased risk of thromboembolic events in the TXA group.[53] The Clinical Randomization of an Antifibrinolytic in Significant Head Injury (CRASH-3) is ongoing (NCT01402882).

TOPICAL HEMOSTATIC AGENTS

Topical hemostatic agents are used as an adjunct to surgical hemostasis when local hemostasis is inadequate. There are 2 types: physical and biological. The latter augments normal hemostasis in the bleeding site and includes fibrin sealant, thrombin gel, and TXA, whereas the physical type activates the local platelet and extrinsic pathway and serve as a scaffold for thrombus formation. In addition, these agents can apply pressure on bleeding vessels. There are limited published data regarding the clinical use of these agents. One of the larger series is a study of 214 patients undergoing cranial or spinal procedures that reported the use of gelatin thrombin hemostatic matrix. All but 11 patients had cessation of bleeding within 3 minutes with no local or systemic complications.[54] The different topical hemostatics and their use in neurosurgical procedures are reviewed by Gazzeri and colleagues.[55] The American Society of Anesthesiology recommends considering the use of topical hemostatics, such as fibrin glue or thrombin, in patients with excessive bleeding.[25]

DESMOPRESSIN

DDAVP stimulates the release of von Willebrand factor from endothelial cells and increases the plasma levels of von Willebrand factor and factor VIII, and it may also increase platelet adhesion molecules. It is routinely used for patients with von Willebrand disease, hemophilia A, and uremia-induced platelet dysfunction. It has been shown in a small prospective trial that DDAVP improved platelet activity after ICH with a reduced rate of hematoma growth in 14 patients of whom 9 were on aspirin.[56] An additional small study reported improved platelet function 30 minutes after DDAVP administration in 13 patients with ICH from a variety of reasons (10 were aspirin users). However, this improvement was short and the platelet function worsened at 3 hours.[57] The Neurocritical Care Society recommends the use of a single dose of DDAVP (0.4 mcg/kg) for ICH associated with aspirin/cyclooxygenase-1 inhibitors or adenosine diphosphate receptor inhibitors.[28] The use of DDAVP for patients without a congenital bleeding disorder or antiplatelet treatment was less clear. In a recently published observational cohort study of 1639 patients with SAH, DDAVP was given to 12% of the patients (0.3 mcg/kg). DDAVP administration was associated with 45% reduction in the risk for rebleeding independent of prior use of antiplatelet agents.[58]

SUMMARY

Adequate hemostasis during neurosurgical procedures is vital for favorable outcomes. Even patients with optimal preparation can have unanticipated severe hemorrhage as well as patients going through emergent/urgent procedure. It is of paramount importance to identify the reason for the bleeding and treat accordingly. The mainstream of treatment remains transfusion of needed cells and factors components (platelets, FFP, RBC, and cryoprecipitate), keeping in mind massive transfusion protocols when needed, and in conjunction with pharmacologic treatment when needed (eg, PCC). It is important to realize that some of the recommendations are extrapolated from ICH or non-neurosurgical data. Patients who did not receive TXA or DDAVP before the surgery might benefit from their administration in the appropriate clinical scenario. Lastly, patients not responding to other measures might benefit from rFVIIa. Ongoing and future clinical trials will better guide us on the specific optimal treatments for subgroups of patients.

REFERENCES

1. Maegele M, Schochl H, Menovsky T, et al. Coagulopathy and haemorrhagic progression in traumatic brain injury: advances in mechanisms, diagnosis, and management. Lancet Neurol 2017;16(8): 630–47.
2. Velez AM, Friedman WA. Disseminated intravascular coagulation during resection of a meningioma: case report. Neurosurgery 2011;68(4):E1165–9 [discussion: E1169].
3. Brecknell JE, McLean CA, Hirano H, et al. Disseminated intravascular coagulation complicating resection of a malignant meningioma. Br J Neurosurg 2006;20(4):239–41.
4. Pinggera D, Kerschbaumer J, Innerhofer N, et al. Disseminated intravascular coagulation in secondary glioblastoma due to excessive intraoperative bleeding: case report and review of the literature. World Neurosurg 2016;90:702.e7-11.
5. Levi M, Toh CH, Thachil J, et al. Guidelines for the diagnosis and management of disseminated intravascular coagulation. British committee for standards in haematology. Br J Haematol 2009;145(1): 24–33.
6. Taylor FB Jr, Toh C-H, Hoots WK, et al. Towards definition, clinical and laboratory criteria, and a scoring system for disseminated intravascular coagulation. On behalf of the Scientific Subcommittee on Disseminated Intravascular Coagulation (DIC) of the ISTH. Thromb Haemost 2001;86(11):1327–30.
7. Bakhtiari K, Meijers JC, de Jonge E, et al. Prospective validation of the international society of thrombosis and haemostasis scoring system for disseminated intravascular coagulation. Crit Care Med 2004;32(12):2416–21.
8. Kvint S, Schuster J, Kumar MA. Neurosurgical applications of viscoelastic hemostatic assays. Neurosurg Focus 2017;43(5):E9.
9. Luostarinen T, Silvasti-Lundell M, Medeiros T, et al. Thromboelastometry during intraoperative transfusion of fresh frozen plasma in pediatric neurosurgery. J Anesth 2012;26(5):770–4.
10. Wikkelso A, Wetterslev J, Moller AM, et al. Thromboelastography (TEG) or rotational thromboelastometry (ROTEM) to monitor haemostatic treatment in bleeding patients: a systematic review with meta-analysis and trial sequential analysis. Anaesthesia 2017;72(4):519–31.
11. Hunt H, Stanworth S, Curry N, et al. Thromboelastography (TEG) and rotational thromboelastometry (ROTEM) for trauma induced coagulopathy in adult trauma patients with bleeding. Cochrane Database Syst Rev 2015;(2):CD010438.
12. Ellenberger C, Garofano N, Barcelos G, et al. Assessment of haemostasis in patients undergoing emergent neurosurgery by rotational elastometry and standard coagulation tests: a prospective observational study. BMC Anesthesiol 2017; 17(1):146.
13. Kozek-Langenecker SA, Afshari A, Albaladejo P, et al. Management of severe perioperative bleeding: guidelines from the European society of anaesthesiology. Eur J Anaesthesiol 2013;30(6):270–382.
14. West KL, Adamson C, Hoffman M. Prophylactic correction of the international normalized ratio in neurosurgery: a brief review of a brief literature. J Neurosurg 2011;114(1):9–18.
15. Kozek-Langenecker SA, Ahmed AB, Afshari A, et al. Management of severe perioperative bleeding: guidelines from the European society of anaesthesiology: first update 2016. Eur J Anaesthesiol 2017; 34(6):332–95.
16. Mangram A, Oguntodu OF, Dzandu JK, et al. Is there a difference in efficacy, safety, and cost-effectiveness between 3-factor and 4-factor prothrombin complex concentrates among trauma

patients on oral anticoagulants? J Crit Care 2016;33: 252–6.

17. Sarode R, Milling TJ Jr, Refaai MA, et al. Efficacy and safety of a 4-factor prothrombin complex concentrate in patients on vitamin K antagonists presenting with major bleeding: a randomized, plasma-controlled, phase IIIb study. Circulation 2013; 128(11):1234–43.

18. Goldstein JN, Refaai MA, Milling TJ Jr, et al. Four-factor prothrombin complex concentrate versus plasma for rapid vitamin K antagonist reversal in patients needing urgent surgical or invasive interventions: a phase 3b, open-label, non-inferiority, randomised trial. Lancet 2015;385(9982):2077–87.

19. Berndtson AE, Huang WT, Box K, et al. A new kid on the block: outcomes with Kcentra 1 year after approval. J Trauma Acute Care Surg 2015;79(6): 1004–8.

20. Beynon C, Nofal M, Rizos T, et al. Anticoagulation reversal with prothrombin complex concentrate in aneurysmal subarachnoid hemorrhage. J Emerg Med 2015;49(5):778–84.

21. Barillari G, Pasca S, Barillari A, et al. Emergency reversal of anticoagulation: from theory to real use of prothrombin complex concentrates. A retrospective Italian experience. Blood Transfus 2012;10(1): 87–94.

22. Beynon C, Potzy A, Unterberg AW, et al. Prothrombin complex concentrate facilitates emergency spinal surgery in anticoagulated patients. Acta Neurochir (Wien) 2014;156(4):741–7.

23. Cartmill M, Dolan G, Byrne JL, et al. Prothrombin complex concentrate for oral anticoagulant reversal in neurosurgical emergencies. Br J Neurosurg 2000;14(5):458–61.

24. Tornkvist M, Smith JG, Labaf A. Current evidence of oral anticoagulant reversal: a systematic review. Thromb Res 2018;162:22–31.

25. American Society of Anesthesiologists Task Force on Perioperative Blood Management. Practice guidelines for perioperative blood management: an updated report by the American society of anesthesiologists task force on perioperative blood management*. Anesthesiology 2015;122(2):241–75.

26. Majeed A, Agren A, Holmstrom M, et al. Management of rivaroxaban- or apixaban-associated major bleeding with prothrombin complex concentrates: a cohort study. Blood 2017;130(15):1706–12.

27. Gerner ST, Kuramatsu JB, Sembill JA, et al. Association of prothrombin complex concentrate administration and hematoma enlargement in non-vitamin K antagonist oral anticoagulant-related intracerebral hemorrhage. Ann Neurol 2018;83(1):186–96.

28. Frontera JA, Lewin JJ 3rd, Rabinstein AA, et al. Guideline for reversal of antithrombotics in intracranial hemorrhage: a statement for healthcare professionals from the neurocritical care society and society of critical care medicine. Neurocrit Care 2016;24(1):6–46.

29. Pollack CV Jr, Reilly PA, van Ryn J, et al. Idarucizumab for dabigatran reversal - full cohort analysis. N Engl J Med 2017;377(5):431–41.

30. Connolly SJ, Milling TJ, Eikelbloom JW, et al. Andexanet for acute major bleeding associated with factor Xa inhibitors. N Engl J Med 2016;375: 1131–41.

31. Bruce D, Nokes TJ. Prothrombin complex concentrate (Beriplex P/N) in severe bleeding: experience in a large tertiary hospital. Crit Care 2008;12(4): R105.

32. Quick JA, Meyer JM, Coughenour JP, et al. Less is more: low-dose prothrombin complex concentrate effective in acute care surgery patients. Am Surg 2015;81(6):646–50.

33. Monroe DM, Hoffman M, Allen GA, et al. The factor VII-platelet interplay: effectiveness of recombinant factor VIIa in the treatment of bleeding in severe thrombocytopathia. Semin Thromb Hemost 2000; 26(4):373–7.

34. Al-Ruzzeh S, Navia JL. The "off-label" role of recombinant factor VIIa in surgery: is the problem deficient evidence or defective concept? J Am Coll Surg 2009;209(5):659–67.

35. Karadimov D, Binev K, Nachkov Y, et al. Use of activated recombinant Factor VII (NovoSeven) during neurosurgery. J Neurosurg Anesthesiol 2003;15(4): 330–2.

36. Kapapa T, Konig K, Heissler HE, et al. The use of recombinant activated factor VII in neurosurgery. Surg Neurol 2009;71(2):172–9 [discussion: 179].

37. Mayer SA, Brun NC, Begtrup K, et al. Efficacy and safety of recombinant activated factor VII for acute intracerebral hemorrhage. N Engl J Med 2008; 358(20):2127–37.

38. Yank V, Tuohy CV, Logan AC, et al. Systematic review: benefits and harms of in-hospital use of recombinant factor VIIa for off-label indications. Ann Intern Med 2011;154(8):529–40.

39. Robinson MT, Rabinstein AA, Meschia JF, et al. Safety of recombinant activated factor VII in patients with warfarin-associated hemorrhages of the central nervous system. Stroke 2010;41(7):1459–63.

40. Yampolsky N, Stofko D, Veznedaroglu E, et al. Recombinant factor VIIa use in patients presenting with intracranial hemorrhage. Springerplus 2014;3:471.

41. Marano G, Vaglio S, Pupella S, et al. How we treat bleeding associated with direct oral anticoagulants. Blood Transfus 2016;14(5):465–73.

42. Schultz NH, Tran HTT, Bjornsen S, et al. The reversal effect of prothrombin complex concentrate (PCC), activated PCC and recombinant activated factor VII against anticoagulation of Xa inhibitor. Thromb J 2017;15:6.

43. Shih AW, Crowther MA. Reversal of direct oral anticoagulants: a practical approach. Hematology Am Soc Hematol Educ Program 2016;2016(1): 612–9.

44. Vermeulen M, Lindsay KW, Murray GD, et al. Antifibrinolytic treatment in subarachnoid hemorrhage. N Engl J Med 1984;311(7):432–7.

45. Hillman J, Fridriksson S, Nilsson O, et al. Immediate administration of tranexamic acid and reduced incidence of early rebleeding after aneurysmal subarachnoid hemorrhage: a prospective randomized study. J Neurosurg 2002;97(4):771–8.

46. Baharoglu MI, Germans MR, Rinkel GJ, et al. Antifibrinolytic therapy for aneurysmal subarachnoid haemorrhage. Cochrane Database Syst Rev 2013;(8): CD001245.

47. Palmer JD, Francis JL, Pickard JD, et al. The efficacy and safety of aprotinin for hemostasis during intracranial surgery. J Neurosurg 2003;98(6): 1208–16.

48. Fergusson DA, Hebert PC, Mazer CD, et al. A comparison of aprotinin and lysine analogues in high-risk cardiac surgery. N Engl J Med 2008; 358(22):2319–31.

49. Mebel D, Akagami R, Flexman AM. Use of tranexamic acid is associated with reduced blood product transfusion in complex skull base neurosurgical procedures: a retrospective cohort study. Anesth Analg 2016;122(2):503–8.

50. Yu CC, Gao WJ, Yang JS, et al. Can tranexamic acid reduce blood loss in cervical laminectomy with lateral mass screw fixation and bone grafting: a retrospective observational study. Medicine (Baltimore) 2017;96(5):e6043.

51. Winter SF, Santaguida C, Wong J, et al. Systemic and topical use of tranexamic acid in spinal surgery: a systematic review. Global Spine J 2016;6(3): 284–95.

52. Perel P, Al-Shahi Salman R, Kawahara T, et al. CRASH-2 (clinical randomisation of an antifibrinolytic in significant haemorrhage) intracranial bleeding study: the effect of tranexamic acid in traumatic brain injury–a nested randomised, placebo-controlled trial. Health Technol Assess 2012;16(13). iii–xii, 1–54.

53. Yutthakasemsunt S, Kittiwatanagul W, Piyavechvirat P, et al. Tranexamic acid for patients with traumatic brain injury: a randomized, double-blinded, placebo-controlled trial. BMC Emerg Med 2013;13:20.

54. Gazzeri R, Galarza M, Neroni M, et al. Hemostatic matrix sealant in neurosurgery: a clinical and imaging study. Acta Neurochir (Wien) 2011;153(1):148–54 [discussion: 155].

55. Gazzeri R, Galarza M, Callovini G, et al. Biosurgical hemostatic agents in neurosurgical intracranial procedures. Surg Technol Int 2017;30:468–76.

56. Naidech AM, Maas MB, Levasseur-Franklin KE, et al. Desmopressin improves platelet activity in acute intracerebral hemorrhage. Stroke 2014;45(8): 2451–3.

57. Kapapa T, Rohrer S, Struve S, et al. Desmopressin acetate in intracranial haemorrhage. Neurol Res Int 2014;2014:298767.

58. Francoeur CL, Roh D, Schmidt JM, et al. Desmopressin administration and rebleeding in subarachnoid hemorrhage: analysis of an observational prospective database. J Neurosurg 2018;1–7. https://doi.org/10.3171/2017.7.JNS17990.

Deep Vein Thrombosis Prophylaxis in the Neurosurgical Patient

Ammar Shaikhouni, MD, PhD*, Justin Baum, MD,
Russell R. Lonser, MD

KEYWORDS

• DVT • PE • DVT prophylaxis

KEY POINTS

- The optimal approach for deep vein thrombosis (DVT) prophylaxis in neurosurgical patients continues to be a challenge of balancing the reduction in DVT and pulmonary embolus (PE) without risking an increase in catastrophic hemorrhages.
- All patients should have mechanical prophylaxis before surgery and continuing after surgery.
- Use of pharmacologic prophylaxis seems to result in an increased rate of hemorrhage in neurosurgery, but weight of the evidence suggests that the addition of pharmacologic prophylaxis reduces the rate of DVT and PE without incurring a high risk of intracerebral hemorrhage once hemostasis is secured and confirmed within 24 to 48 hours after surgery.

CAUSE

Deep vein thrombosis (DVT) is the result of a complex interplay of multiple inherited or acquired factors. The interplay of these factors is summarized using the "Virchow's triad," which includes disturbances in blood flow patterns, blood clotting factors promoting coagulation, and vessel wall endothelial injury. These elements combine to disrupt the balance of coagulation and fibrinolysis mechanisms leading to venous clot formation and propagation.[1] Specifically, the intact endothelium of blood vessel plays an important role in maintaining hemostasis and preventing the formation of clots. Injury to the endothelium of blood vessels, for example, during surgery or with insertion of central venous catheters, exposes subendothelial tissue factor and reduces venous flow, which activates the clotting cascade resulting in thrombus formation.[2]

DVT can form without evidence of injury to the endothelium[3] when stasis and flow turbulence occur in the valve pockets of deep veins.[3–5] These changes lead to local hypoxia that promotes thrombosis by inhibiting expression of anticoagulants and stimulating expression of prothrombotic substances.[6] Acquired factors that promote stasis, such as prolonged immobility, venous valve dysfunction with aging, or increased venous pressure due to heart failure, increase the risk of DVT formation. Similarly, inherited or acquired factors that increase the level/activity of procoagulant or decrease the level/activity of anticoagulants also increase the risk of DVT formation.[2,4–6]

EPIDEMIOLOGY
General Population

Overall estimates for incidence of DVT in the general population range from 45 to 117 per 100,000 persons. DVT formation rates are higher for men (130 per 100,000 persons) than women (110 per 100,000) in all age groups except during the

Disclosure Statement: The authors have nothing to disclose.
Department of Neurological Surgery, Ohio State University Wexner Medical Center, Ohio State University, 410 West 10th Avenue, Columbus, OH 43210, USA
* Corresponding author.
E-mail address: ammar.shaikhouni@osumc.edu

Neurosurg Clin N Am 29 (2018) 567–574
https://doi.org/10.1016/j.nec.2018.06.010

childbearing years (when women are at higher risk). Incidence per 100,000 is highest among African Americans (141) compared with Caucasians (104), Hispanics (55), whereas Asian/Pacific Islanders (21) have the lowest incidence.[7] Age is associated with increased risk of DVT (related to venous valve dysfunction that occurs with aging) development in both men and women.[8] The reported incidence of DVTs has increased with the rising use of routine diagnostic imaging.[8,9]

Neurosurgical Patients

The rate of DVT formation in neurosurgical patients without prophylaxis varies between 0% and 34%.[10–15] Neurosurgical patients receiving at least one form of DVT prophylaxis who underwent screening (asymptomatic) with Doppler ultrasound had a 3% to 16% incidence of DVTs.[16–18] Reported rates of symptomatic DVTs from pooled studies and national databases range between 1% and 4%.[19–22] Differences in reported DVT formation in neurosurgical patients are primarily due to the use and method of screening to detect DVT. Higher-intensity screening has led to higher estimates of DVTs (eg, routine screening of asymptomatic patients). Studies reporting higher rates of DVT used routine screening with high sensitivity tests, such as radioactive fibrinogen uptake, compared with the use of Doppler ultrasound screening of symptomatic patients.[14,23,24]

The risk of DVT formation is associated with neurosurgical procedure location, surgical features, and patient characteristics. Rates are higher for patients undergoing craniotomy compared with spine surgery. Analysis of the National Surgical Quality Improvement Program database (2006–2011) revealed DVT formation was 3.4% after cranial and 1.1% after spinal surgeries.[19,25] Estimates of the incidence of symptomatic DVT from regional hospital discharges reveal a rate of 3.9% for craniotomy patients[26] and a rate of 0.5% to 2% over the 90 days after discharge for the spinal surgery patient.[27] Specifically, among patients undergoing cranial procedures for tumor, the rate of DVT formation was 2% to 10%.[26,28,29] DVT formation in subarachnoid hemorrhage patients ranges between 3.5% and 18%.[20,30,31] The rate of DVT after deep brain stimulation surgery has been reported at 1%.[32] Risk of DVT after surgery for spine trauma, deformity, and degenerative spine surgery is between 0% and 19%, 2% and 14%, and 0% and 9%.[33,34] Patients undergoing a cranial procedure are considered a high- to very high-risk population, whereas patients undergoing spine procedure are considerate a low- to moderate-risk population by the American College of Chest Physicians (ACCP).[35]

Risk factors associated with DVT formation in the neurosurgical patients also include the presence of malignancy, prior episode of DVT and pulmonary embolus (PE), type of surgery (cranial, spinal, or cerebrovascular), duration of surgery, oral contraceptive use, stroke, sepsis, heart failure, radiation therapy, paraparesis, altered mental status, heart failure, smoking, obesity, presence of deep venous catheters, age, and inherited hypercoagulable disorders.[16,19,25,35,36] Risk factors specific for patients undergoing spine surgery include combined anterior-posterior approaches, multilevel surgeries, surgery for trauma, and surgery for deformity correction.[33,35]

PULMONARY EMBOLUS IN THE NEUROSURGICAL PATIENT

PE can result after a DVT travels to the lung vasculature resulting in incomplete or complete blockage of the pulmonary artery (**Fig. 1**). PE is associated with a high rate of morbidity and mortality in the neurosurgical population. Signs and symptoms of PE include tachycardia, pleuritic chest pain, shortness of breath, hemoptysis, and tachypnea. The most severe cases of PE present with sudden cardiopulmonary arrest. Approximately 25% of patients who develop a PE die suddenly. Patients (75% of all PE patients) who survive the acute impact of PE have a 7-day survival rate of 70%.[16] A comprehensive review of the literature estimated the overall rate of PE in neurosurgical patients (patient receiving or not

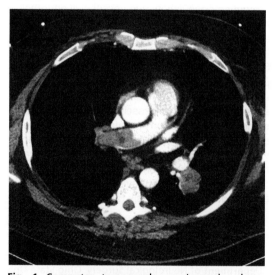

Fig. 1. Computer tomography angiography shows bilateral acute PE (*red star*) in a patient who underwent craniotomy for cranial metastasis removal a few weeks earlier. This patient was also found to have bilateral DVTs in Doppler ultrasound.

receiving prophylaxis) between 0% and 5% with associated mortalities ranging from 9% to 50%.[37] Large single-center studies of neurosurgical patients that received either mechanical prophylaxis with or without pharmacologic prophylaxis report an incidence of PE of 0.3% to 0.8% with an associated mortality of 0% to 18%.[16,38] Estimates using pooled studies' data and national databases estimate the rate of PE to be approximately half of symptomatic DVT, ranging from 0.4% to 1.2%.[19–22,25]

DEEP VEIN THROMBOSIS PROPHYLAXIS IN THE NEUROSURGICAL PATIENT
General

DVT is the underlying cause of PE in approximately 36% to 45% of cases.[36] Because of the role of DVT in PE and the high mortality associated with PE, it is critical to implement methods to prevent DVT.[16,35,39] The most commonly used DVT prophylaxis methods in neurosurgical patients are mechanical, pharmacologic, or a combination of these 2 methods.[36,39,40]

Mechanical Prophylaxis

The most common mechanical methods for DVT prophylaxis are compression stockings (CS) and intermittent pneumatic compression (IPC) of the lower extremities. Both CS and IPC are thought to reduce the incidence of DVTs by enhancing blood flow in the lower extremities and reducing venous stasis. CS compress veins and reduce their diameter, which in turn increases blood flow velocity.[41] IPC devices enhance the effect of compression by using a pump to inflate and deflate cuffs wrapped around extremities. Increased blood flow velocity through these vessels decreases the amount of blood products that accumulate and lead to clot formation, ultimately reducing DVT.[42] Moreover, IPC enhances fibrinolytic activity by reducing the activity of plasminogen activator inhibitor function with a resulting increase in the activity of tissue plasminogen activator.[43]

CS and IPC devices are effective. They have been shown to decrease the relative risk of DVTs in postsurgical patients by 50% to 60%.[44–48] Studies in the neurosurgical population are limited but show a reduction in risk of DVTs versus placebo (relative risk ratio 0.41; range 0.21–0.78).[15] Although no definitive studies exist comparing ICD directly to CS (in isolation), there is evidence indicating that IPC may offer superior protection to CS alone.[49] The risks of IPCs and CSs are minimal and include discomfort and skin breakdown. Although CS are easy to apply,

IPC devices suffer from poor patient compliance, poor fitting, and common application errors.[50] IPCs are contraindicated in patients with leg ischemia.[41] Mechanical prophylaxis is strongly recommended by the ACCP for cranial and spinal neurosurgery.[35]

Pharmacologic Prophylaxis

The 2 most common pharmacologic prophylaxis agents include low-dose unfractionated heparin (UFH) and low-molecular-weight heparin (LMWH). Natural heparin consists of various molecules of differing lengths, which can cause different therapeutic effects. UFH is a polyglycosaminoglycan that binds to thrombin (factor IIa) and factor Xa. Because of its molecular weight, UFH preferentially binds to factor IIa. LMWHs are short chains of heparin that are obtained by "fractionating" natural heparin. These shorter chains bind selectively to factor Xa. UFH has a half-life of 90 minutes, whereas LMWH's half-life is approximately 4 hours. LMWHs have been shown to be more predictable than UFH in producing anticoagulation effects.[51,52]

Prospective randomized studies examining chemoprophylaxis alone in neurosurgical patients have resulted in differing conclusions. Cerrato and colleagues[13] randomized 100 patients to receive 5000 units of subcutaneous heparin beginning 2 hours before brain tumor surgery and every 8 hours thereafter versus receive no prophylaxis. They found subcutaneous heparin significantly decreased postoperative DVT formation from 34% to 6% compared with controls. Constantini and colleagues[53] studied 103 patients undergoing resection of supratentorial brain tumors. They randomized their patients to receive 5000 units of subcutaneous heparin 2 hours before surgery and every 12 hours thereafter or receive no prophylaxis. There was no significant difference in DVT formation (2 patients in each group developed DVTs).

There are 2 small studies that compared the use of low-dose UFH with LMWH.[54,55] Neither study has shown that one agent is superior to the other in terms of efficacy or safety. Investigators who argue for the use of LMWH cite its more predictable pharmacology and reported lower risk of hemorrhage in other patient populations.[14,54–56] The current data do not offer definite support for the use of one agent over the other. However, in certain patient populations, such as patients with severe renal failure wherein the dosing of LMWH is not well defined, it is better to use low-dose UFH to avoid the underdosing or overdosing of heparin.[57]

A major risk for pharmacologic prophylaxis against DVTs is hemorrhage. Dickinson and colleagues[58] studied the safety of LMWH compared with IPC devices. The study was terminated early because 5 out of 46 patients receiving LMWH suffered from clinically significant intracranial hemorrhage compared with none in the IPC group. Although pooled data analysis by Collen and colleagues[15] showed a rate of major postoperative hemorrhage of 0.04% for IPC, 0.35% for UFH, and 1.52% for LMWH, none of the differences were significant. Heparin-induced thrombocytopenia is another potential complication of chemical prophylaxis due to an immune reaction against platelet factor IV in complex with heparin. It occurs in less than 5% of patients exposed to heparin.[59] It is more commonly observed with UFH (2.6%) than with LMWH (0.2%).[60] Treatment requires the cessation of the heparin and use of alternative anticoagulants along with supportive therapy.

Combination of Mechanical and Chemical Prophylaxis

Because mechanical and chemical prophylaxis inhibits clot formation by different pathways, the use of both may synergistically decrease DVT formation. Two randomized trials compared combination of IPC and LMWH versus IPC alone in a general neurosurgical patient population and found significant decrease in rate of any (symptomatic and asymptomatic) DVTs and PEs in the IPC and LMWH group. Both studies also reported a nonsignificant increase in the rate of major bleeding complications in the IPC and LMWH group.[14,61] This result was confirmed by multiple other larger single-institution mixed neurosurgical population retrospective chart reviews.[16,62] Both retrospective and prospective studies comparing pharmacologic and mechanical prophylaxis to mechanical prophylaxis in spine-only patients showed a decreased rate of DVT/PE and an increase in the rate of major hemorrhage in the combination group compared with the mechanical prophylaxis group only, but neither were statistically significant.[33,63,64]

Meta-analyses, although limited by heterogeneity of studies, can overcome the limitations of small studies by data pooling. Four meta-analyses address DVT prophylaxis in neurosurgery. A large meta-analysis by Collen and colleagues[15] concluded that use of IPC devices or heparin prophylaxis was effective in reducing the rate of DVTs compared with no prophylaxis, but there was no significant difference between rate of DVTs or major hemorrhages in patients treated with IPC devices, heparin, or a combination of the 2. Alternatively, Iorio and Agnelli[24] found that heparin prophylaxis led to a 45% or 50% relative risk reduction of total and proximal DVTs compared with nonpharmacologic prophylaxis methods with a statistically insignificant 71% increase in relative risk of major hemorrhage. Hamilton and colleagues[56] found that heparin (in craniotomy patients) is protective whether used alone or with the addition of mechanical prophylaxis compared with mechanical prophylaxis alone. There was a higher statistically nonsignificant incidence of intracerebral hemorrhage (ICH) in the heparin-treated group compared with the non-heparin-treated group. The most recent meta-analysis included 9 studies looking at DVT prophylaxis in neurosurgical (including cranial and spinal procedures) patients. They calculated an absolute risk reduction of 9% of DVT formation and a relative risk reduction of 42% in the patients treated with pharmacologic prophylaxis (either UFH or LMWH) versus control (analysis of 1232 patients). There was no significant difference in intracranial hemorrhage rates in cranial surgery patients (2.7% in the chemoprophylaxis group vs 1.6% in the control groups) and no significant difference in hemorrhagic complications in spinal surgery patients.[65]

Prophylactic Paradigms

Mechanical methods of DVT prophylaxis in neurosurgical patients have been shown to be an effective and safe method for DVT prophylaxis and should be used in neurosurgical patients, as recommended by the ACCP.[35] The addition of a pharmacologic agent to mechanical prophylaxis requires balancing the benefit of DVT/PE prevention with increased risk of hemorrhage. The ACCP guidelines recommend avoiding the use of pharmacologic prophylaxis for patients with low risk of DVT/PE and to recommend the use of pharmacologic prophylaxis in patients with high risk of DVT/PE once "adequate hemostasis is established, and risk of bleeding decreases."[35] The North American Spine Society recommends use of mechanical prophylaxis only for patients undergoing elective spine procedures and recommends the careful consideration of the addition of heparin to mechanical prophylaxis in patients undergoing spine surgery for trauma, deformity, or malignancy.[66]

The above recommendation reflects the unavailability of high-quality large randomized studies to help guide decision making regarding the best DVT prophylaxis strategy that balances the risk-reward ratio of lowering DVT/PE without increasing catastrophic hemorrhages. Because such studies are unlikely to be completed, some suggested the use of computer simulation studies to explore prophylaxis strategies. Danish and colleagues[21] calculated the incidence of DVTs and PEs in neurosurgical patients treated using IPCs alone or in combination with UFH or LMWH using a weighted average of pooled data from multiple studies. Based on these data, they concluded that the most effective method of prophylaxis (balancing the rates of morbidity and mortality from DVT/PE and ICH) in craniotomy patients is mechanical compression only. The addition of UFC to mechanical prophylaxis becomes effective once the risk of PE approaches 1.4%. However, a similar analysis by Algattas and colleagues[67] concluded that UFH and mechanical prophylaxis were more cost-effective than mechanical prophylaxis and LMWH or mechanical prophylaxis alone. Both studies are biased by the assumption of utility and cost of DVT, PE, and ICH.

If the decision is made to add pharmacologic prophylaxis to mechanical prophylaxis, the next question to answer is, what is the safe time to initiate it? Pharmacologic prophylaxis studies have begun chemoprophylaxis either within 24 hours after surgery or at various intervals before surgery.[39] Although most of these studies did not find any statistically significant increase in bleeding risk in the chemoprophylaxis-treated patients, the investigators who did report increased bleeding risks were in patients who received chemoprophylaxis preoperatively. In comprehensive reviews of the literature, rates of ICH in patients who preoperatively received 5000 units of subcutaneous heparin either 2 or 3 times daily ranged between 1.3% and 5.2% compared with 2% to 4.3% in patients who did not receive heparin.[39] Lower rates of ICH are reported when heparin is given postoperatively and range between 0% and 1.8%.[62,68] Khaldi and colleagues[16] administered subcutaneous heparin either 24 or 48 hours postoperatively and showed a similar decrease in rate of asymptomatic DVT without an increase in rate of hemorrhage. Based on the culmination of the previous studies, it feasible to initiate mechanical prophylaxis in the neurosurgery patient before surgery and add chemoprophylaxis 24 hours after surgery to reduce the reported increased risk in hemorrhage when heparin was started preoperatively.

Pediatric Patients

The incidence of DVT/PE among pediatric patients is exceedingly rare. Tabori and colleagues[69] studied the incidence of DVT among pediatric patients with brain tumors and found that only 0.64% of children with brain tumor experience clinically significant DVT/PE. Gonda and colleagues[70] investigated the use of LMWH for prophylaxis in 24 children admitted to neurosurgical service and found a rate of ICH in treated patients of 4% (1 patient). Although this 1 patient had other bleeding risk factors, the above results have been taken to suggest that pediatric patients are more likely to be harmed by pharmacologic DVT prophylaxis than helped because of the low risk of DVT in this population. Furthermore, providing an accurate dose of pharmacologic agent in the pediatric population is difficult because of variation in the size of children, therefore risking underdosing or overdosing the medication. These findings have led many to avoid DVT prophylaxis for pediatric patients until more data become available about the rate of DVT/PEs and risks of DVT prophylaxis in this population.

SUMMARY

Data in neurosurgical patients show that the addition of pharmacologic prophylaxis to mechanical prophylaxis results in a decrease in the rate of DVTs along with a possible increase in incidence of hemorrhages. Reported data are currently not sufficient to accurately weigh the risk of increased hemorrhage compared with the benefit of reduction of DVT and/or PE.

REFERENCES

1. Kumar DR, Hanlin E, Glurich I, et al. Virchow's contribution to the understanding of thrombosis and cellular biology. Clin Med Res 2010;8(3–4): 168–72.
2. Turpie AGG, Esmon C. Venous and arterial thrombosis – pathogenesis and the rationale for anticoagulation. Thromb Haemost 2011;105(04):586–96.
3. Sevitt S. The structure and growth of valve-pocket thrombi in femoral veins. J Clin Pathol 1974;27(7): 517–28.
4. Stone J, Hangge P, Albadawi H, et al. Deep vein thrombosis: pathogenesis, diagnosis, and medical management. Cardiovasc Diagn Ther 2017; 7(Suppl 3):S276–84.
5. Esmon CT. Basic mechanisms and pathogenesis of venous thrombosis. Blood Rev 2009;23(5):225–9.
6. Bovill EG, van der Vliet A. Venous valvular stasis–associated hypoxia and thrombosis: what is the link? Annu Rev Physiol 2011;73(1):527–45.
7. Keenan CR, White RH. The effects of race/ethnicity and sex on the risk of venous thromboembolism. Curr Opin Pulm Med 2007;13(5):377–83.
8. Heit JA. Epidemiology of venous thromboembolism. Nat Rev Cardiol 2015;12(8):464–74.

9. Huang W, Goldberg RJ, Anderson FA, et al. Secular trends in occurrence of acute venous thromboembolism: the Worcester VTE study (1985-2009). Am J Med 2014;127(9):829–39.e5.

10. Turpie AG, Gallus A, Beattie WS, et al. Prevention of venous thrombosis in patients with intracranial disease by intermittent pneumatic compression of the calf. Neurology 1977;27(5):435–8.

11. Turpie AG, Hirsh J, Gent M, et al. Prevention of deep vein thrombosis in potential neurosurgical patients. A randomized trial comparing graduated compression stockings alone or graduated compression stockings plus intermittent pneumatic compression with control. Arch Intern Med 1989;149(3):679–81.

12. Boström S, Holmgren E, Jonsson O, et al. Post-operative thromboembolism in neurosurgery. A study on the prophylactic effect of calf muscle stimulation plus dextran compared to low-dose heparin. Acta Neurochir (Wien) 1986;80(3–4):83–9.

13. Cerrato D, Ariano C, Fiacchino F. Deep vein thrombosis and low-dose heparin prophylaxis in neurosurgical patients. J Neurosurg 1978;49(3):378–81.

14. Agnelli G, Piovella F, Buoncristiani P, et al. Enoxaparin plus compression stockings compared with compression stockings alone in the prevention of venous thromboembolism after elective neurosurgery. N Engl J Med 1998;339(2):80–5.

15. Collen JF, Jackson JL, Shorr AF, et al. Prevention of venous thromboembolism in neurosurgery: a metaanalysis. Chest 2008;134(2):237–49.

16. Khaldi A, Helo N, Schneck MJ, et al. Venous thromboembolism: deep venous thrombosis and pulmonary embolism in a neurosurgical population. J Neurosurg 2010;114(1):40–6.

17. Patel SR, Sheth SA, Mian MK, et al. Single-neuron responses in the human nucleus accumbens during a financial decision-making task. J Neurosci 2012;32(21):7311–5.

18. Henwood PC, Kennedy TM, Thomson L, et al. The incidence of deep vein thrombosis detected by routine surveillance ultrasound in neurosurgery patients receiving dual modality prophylaxis. J Thromb Thrombolysis 2011;32(2):209–14.

19. Rolston JD, Han SJ, Bloch O, et al. What clinical factors predict the incidence of deep venous thrombosis and pulmonary embolism in neurosurgical patients? J Neurosurg 2014;121(4):908–18.

20. Kshettry VR, Rosenbaum BP, Seicean A, et al. Incidence and risk factors associated with in-hospital venous thromboembolism after aneurysmal subarachnoid hemorrhage. J Clin Neurosci 2014;21(2):282–6.

21. Danish SF, Burnett MG, Ong JG, et al. Prophylaxis for deep venous thrombosis in craniotomy patients: a decision analysis. Neurosurgery 2005;56(6):1286–92 [discussion: 1292–4].

22. Kimmell KT, Jahromi BS. Clinical factors associated with venous thromboembolism risk in patients undergoing craniotomy. J Neurosurg 2015;122(5):1004–11.

23. Ganau M, Prisco L, Cebula H, et al. Risk of deep vein thrombosis in neurosurgery: state of the art on prophylaxis protocols and best clinical practices. J Clin Neurosci 2017;45:60–6.

24. Iorio A, Agnelli G. Low-molecular-weight and unfractionated heparin for prevention of venous thromboembolism in neurosurgery: a meta-analysis. Arch Intern Med 2000;160(15):2327–32.

25. Piper K, Algattas H, DeAndrea-Lazarus IA, et al. Risk factors associated with venous thromboembolism in patients undergoing spine surgery. J Neurosurg Spine 2017;26(1):90–6.

26. Chan AT, Atiemo A, Diran LK, et al. Venous thromboembolism occurs frequently in patients undergoing brain tumor surgery despite prophylaxis. J Thromb Thrombolysis 1999;8(2):139–42.

27. White RH, Zhou H, Romano PS. Incidence of symptomatic venous thromboembolism after different elective or urgent surgical procedures. Thromb Haemost 2003;90(3):446–55.

28. Cote DJ, Dubois HM, Karhade AV, et al. Venous thromboembolism in patients undergoing craniotomy for brain tumors: a U.S. nationwide analysis. Semin Thromb Hemost 2016;42(8):870–6.

29. Senders JT, Goldhaber NH, Cote DJ, et al. Venous thromboembolism and intracranial hemorrhage after craniotomy for primary malignant brain tumors: a National Surgical Quality Improvement Program analysis. J Neurooncol 2018;136(1):135–45.

30. Ray WZ, Strom RG, Blackburn SL, et al. Incidence of deep venous thrombosis after subarachnoid hemorrhage. J Neurosurg 2009;110(5):1010–4.

31. Serrone JC, Wash EM, Hartings JA, et al. Venous thromboembolism in subarachnoid hemorrhage. World Neurosurg 2013;80(6):859–63.

32. Bauman JA, Church E, Halpern CH, et al. Subcutaneous heparin for prophylaxis of venous thromboembolism in deep brain stimulation surgeryevidence from a decision analysis. Neurosurgery 2009;65(2):276–80.

33. Cheng JS, Arnold PM, Anderson PA, et al. Anticoagulation risk in spine surgery. Spine 2010;35(9 Suppl):S117–24.

34. Glotzbecker MP, Bono CM, Wood KB, et al. Thromboembolic disease in spinal surgery: a systematic review. Spine 2009;34(3):291–303.

35. Gould MK, Garcia DA, Wren SM, et al. Prevention of VTE in nonorthopedic surgical patients: antithrombotic therapy and prevention of thrombosis, 9th ed: American College of Chest Physicians Evidence-Based Clinical Practice Guidelines. Chest 2012;141(2 Suppl):e227S–77S.

36. Epstein NE. A review of the risks and benefits of differing prophylaxis regimens for the treatment of deep venous thrombosis and pulmonary embolism in neurosurgery. Surg Neurol 2005;64(4):295–301.

37. Hamilton MG, Hull RD, Pineo GF. Venous thromboembolism in neurosurgery and neurology patients: a review. Neurosurgery 1994;34(2):280–96 [discussion: 296].

38. Patel AP, Koltz MT, Sansur CA, et al. An analysis of deep vein thrombosis in 1277 consecutive neurosurgical patients undergoing routine weekly ultrasonography. J Neurosurg 2013;118(3):505–9.

39. Browd SR, Ragel BT, Davis GE, et al. Prophylaxis for deep venous thrombosis in neurosurgery: a review of the literature. Neurosurg Focus 2004;17(4):E1.

40. Gnanalingham KK, Holland JP. Attitudes to the use of prophylaxis for thrombo-embolism in neurosurgical patients. J Clin Neurosci 2003;10(4):467–9.

41. Lim CS, Davies AH. Graduated compression stockings. CMAJ 2014;186(10):E391–8.

42. Roberts VC, Sabri S, Beeley AH, et al. The effect of intermittently applied external pressure on the haemodynamics of the lower limb in man. Br J Surg 1972;59(3):223–6.

43. Comerota AJ, Chouhan V, Harada RN, et al. The fibrinolytic effects of intermittent pneumatic compression: mechanism of enhanced fibrinolysis. Ann Surg 1997;226(3):306–14.

44. Roderick P, Ferris G, Wilson K, et al. Towards evidence-based guidelines for the prevention of venous thromboembolism: systematic reviews of mechanical methods, oral anticoagulation, dextran and regional anaesthesia as thromboprophylaxis. Health Technol Assess 2005;9(49). iii–iv, ix–x, 1–78.

45. Ho KM, Tan JA. Stratified meta-analysis of intermittent pneumatic compression of the lower limbs to prevent venous thromboembolism in hospitalized patientsclinical perspective. Circulation 2013;128(9):1003–20.

46. Wells PS, Lensing AW, Hirsh J. Graduated compression stockings in the prevention of postoperative venous thromboembolism. A meta-analysis. Arch Intern Med 1994;154(1):67–72.

47. Agu O, Hamilton G, Baker D. Graduated compression stockings in the prevention of venous thromboembolism. Br J Surg 1999;86(8):992–1004.

48. Urbankova J, Quiroz R, Kucher N, et al. Intermittent pneumatic compression and deep vein thrombosis prevention. A meta-analysis in postoperative patients. Thromb Haemost 2005;94(6):1181–5.

49. Prell J, Schenk G, Taute B-M, et al. Reduced risk of venous thromboembolism with the use of intermittent pneumatic compression after craniotomy: a randomized controlled prospective study. J Neurosurg 2018;1–7. [Epub ahead of print].

50. Elpern E, Killeen K, Patel G, et al. The application of intermittent pneumatic compression devices for thromboprophylaxis: an observational study found frequent errors in the application of these mechanical devices in icus. Am J Nurs 2013;113(4):30–6 [quiz: 37].

51. Hirsh J, Warkentin TE, Shaughnessy SG, et al. Heparin and low-molecular-weight heparin mechanisms of action, pharmacokinetics, dosing, monitoring, efficacy, and safety. Chest 2001;119(1, Supplement):64S–94S.

52. Adler BK. Unfractionated heparin and other antithrombin mediated anticoagulants. Clin Lab Sci 2004;17(2):113–7.

53. Constantini S, Kanner A, Friedman A, et al. Safety of perioperative minidose heparin in patients undergoing brain tumor surgery: a prospective, randomized, double-blind study. J Neurosurg 2001;94(6):918–21.

54. Macdonald RL, Amidei C, Baron J, et al. Randomized, pilot study of intermittent pneumatic compression devices plus dalteparin versus intermittent pneumatic compression devices plus heparin for prevention of venous thromboembolism in patients undergoing craniotomy. Surg Neurol 2003;59(5):362–71.

55. Goldhaber SZ, Dunn K, Gerhard-Herman M, et al. Low rate of venous thromboembolism after craniotomy for brain tumor using multimodality prophylaxis. Chest 2002;122(6):1933–7.

56. Hamilton MG, Yee WH, Hull RD, et al. Venous thromboembolism prophylaxis in patients undergoing cranial neurosurgery: a systematic review and meta-analysis. Neurosurgery 2011;68(3):571–81.

57. Nutescu EA, Spinler SA, Wittkowsky A, et al. Low-molecular-weight heparins in renal impairment and obesity: available evidence and clinical practice recommendations across medical and surgical settings. Ann Pharmacother 2009;43(6):1064–83.

58. Dickinson LD, Miller LD, Patel CP, et al. Enoxaparin increases the incidence of postoperative intracranial hemorrhage when initiated preoperatively for deep venous thrombosis prophylaxis in patients with brain tumors. Neurosurgery 1998;43(5):1074–81.

59. Ahmed I, Majeed A, Powell R. Heparin induced thrombocytopenia: diagnosis and management update. Postgrad Med J 2007;83(983):575–82.

60. Martel N, Lee J, Wells PS. Risk for heparin-induced thrombocytopenia with unfractionated and low-molecular-weight heparin thromboprophylaxis: a meta-analysis. Blood 2005;106(8):2710–5.

61. Nurmohamed MT, van Riel AM, Henkens CM, et al. Low molecular weight heparin and compression stockings in the prevention of venous thromboembolism in neurosurgery. Thromb Haemost 1996;75(2):233–8.

62. Frim DM, Barker FG, Poletti CE, et al. Postoperative low-dose heparin decreases thromboembolic complications in neurosurgical patients. Neurosurgery 1992;30(6):830–2 [discussion: 832–3].

63. Hamidi S, Riazi M. Incidence of venous thromboembolic complications in instrumental spinal surgeries with preoperative chemoprophylaxis. J Korean Neurosurg Soc 2015;57(2):114–8.

64. Mosenthal WP, Landy DC, Boyajian HH, et al. Thromboprophylaxis in spinal surgery. Spine (Phila Pa 1976) 2018;43(8):E474–81.

65. Khan NR, Patel PG, Sharpe JP, et al. Chemical venous thromboembolism prophylaxis in neurosurgical patients: an updated systematic review and meta-analysis. J Neurosurg 2017;1–10. https://doi.org/10.3171/2017.2.JNS162040.

66. Bono CM, Watters WC, Heggeness MH, et al. An evidence-based clinical guideline for the use of antithrombotic therapies in spine surgery. Spine J 2009;9(12):1046–51.

67. Algattas H, Damania D, DeAndrea-Lazarus I, et al. Systematic review of safety and cost-effectiveness of venous thromboembolism prophylaxis strategies in patients undergoing craniotomy for brain tumor. Neurosurgery 2018;82(2):142–54.

68. Raabe A, Gerlach R, Zimmermann M, et al. The risk of haemorrhage associated with early postoperative heparin administration after intracranial surgery. Acta Neurochir (Wien) 2001;143(1):1–7.

69. Tabori U, Beni-Adani L, Dvir R, et al. Risk of venous thromboembolism in pediatric patients with brain tumors. Pediatr Blood Cancer 2004;43(6):633–6.

70. Gonda DD, Fridley J, Ryan SL, et al. The safety and efficacy of use of low-molecular-weight heparin in pediatric neurosurgical patients. J Neurosurg Pediatr 2015;16(3):329–34.

Postoperative Anticoagulation After Neurologic Surgery

Joel Z. Passer, MD[a], Christopher M. Loftus, MD[b],*

KEYWORDS

- Anticoagulation • Antiplatelet • Atrial fibrillation • Mechanical heart valve • VTE • Stent-coil
- Pipeline • Intrathecal access

KEY POINTS

- Reinitiation of antiplatelet and anticoagulant medications after neurosurgery is complex, but the process can be aided by scoring systems to stratify the risk/benefit ratio.
- Most neurosurgical patients are at high risk of postoperative venous thromboembolism.
- Appropriate prophylaxis with pneumatic compression devices, graduated compression stockings and pharmacologic prophylaxis can significantly decrease complication rates.
- Management of antiplatelet medications before and after placement of neuroendovascular devices can be aided with the use of readily available platelet function assays. Patients can experience significant resistance or responsiveness to these medications.
- Placement of intrathecal access devices (ventricular drain, lumbar puncture or lumbar drain catheter) in the setting of antiplatelet or anticoagulant medications can be dangerous, but can be done safely using proper precautions.

INTRODUCTION

Neurosurgeons are performing more procedures on a wide variety of patients, many of whom are advanced in age and have multiple medical comorbidities. These multifactorial medical issues may necessitate the use of anticoagulant or antiplatelet medications, of which use has increased in the United States in recent years.[1,2] In addition, there are neurosurgical conditions and devices that necessitate the use of these medications as part of the treatment algorithm.[3]

The debate as when to reinstitute postoperatively or, in some cases, begin treatment with preoperatively these medications has been a long-standing debate in the field. A balance must exist between preventing venous thromboembolism (VTE), pulmonary embolism (PE) and ischemic stroke, with preventing postoperative hematoma in the surgical bed. This review seeks to elucidate how to best reinitiate anticoagulation therapy for patients after neurosurgical procedures and intracranial hemorrhage (ICH), demonstrates appropriate management of antiplatelet therapy after placement of neuroendovascular devices, reviews postoperative initiation of VTE prophylaxis and treatment modalities, and reviews the safety of cerebrospinal fluid access procedures (ventricular drain, lumbar puncture, lumbar drain) on patients taking anticoagulation or antiplatelet therapy.

Disclosure Statement: The authors have nothing to disclose.
[a] Department of Neurosurgery, Temple University Hospital, 3401 North Broad Street, Suite C540, Philadelphia, PA 19140, USA; [b] Department of Neurosurgery, Lewis Katz School of Medicine, Temple University, Temple University Hospital, 3401 North Broad Street, Suite C540, Philadelphia, PA 19140, USA
* Corresponding author.
E-mail address: christopher.loftus@tuhs.temple.edu

Neurosurg Clin N Am 29 (2018) 575–583
https://doi.org/10.1016/j.nec.2018.06.008
1042-3680/18/© 2018 Elsevier Inc. All rights reserved.

PATIENTS WITH STRUCTURAL DISEASE WHO NEED ANTICOAGULATION

Atrial Fibrillation

Atrial fibrillation (AF) is the most common cardiac arrhythmia in the elderly and millions of people in the United States have been diagnosed with AF, with incidence expected to increase in the coming years.[4] One of the principal complications of AF is ischemic stroke. Assessment of risk of stroke in nonvalvular AF has been validated with multiple scoring systems, including $CHADS_2$ and its more updated counterpart, CHA_2DS_2VASc. These scoring systems account for congestive heart failure, hypertension, age greater than 75 years, diabetes mellitus, history of prior stroke or transient ischemic attack, and additionally in CHA_2DS_2-VASc: history of vascular disease, age between 64 to 75 years, and sex (female gender). This scoring system gives 1 point for presence of each risk factor (2 points for history of previous stroke/transient ischemic attack or age >75 years) and the total score corresponds with a percent annual stroke risk, with higher scores having higher annual risk of stroke. Patients with a score of 2 or greater have been shown to be at high risk of stroke (2.2% risk for a score of 2, with risk increasing for each additional point) and are recommended to take oral anticoagulation using either a vitamin K antagonist, such as warfarin, or a novel oral anticoagulant (NOAC) on the basis of guidelines from the American College of Cardiology/American Heart Association and the European Society of Cardiology.[5,6] In early trials, warfarin was shown to prevent stroke in AF compared with placebo/aspirin, with a decrease from 4.5% to 1.4% annually. Inversely, the risk of hemorrhage on warfarin therapy is increased and rates of major hemorrhage historically were 1.3% versus 1% on placebo/aspirin.[7]

Warfarin use in AF is complex. Owing to concern for hemorrhage on warfarin therapy as well as need for monitoring of International Normalized Ratio levels at least once weekly during initiation, as well as once monthly when stabilized,[5] NOACs have been developed as a potentially safer and simpler alternative. Dabigatran is a direct thrombin inhibitor approved by the US Food and Drug Administration in 2010 for the prevention of stroke and systemic embolism in patients with nonvalvular AF. The Randomized Evaluation of Long-Term Anticoagulation Therapy (RE-LY) trial showed that dabigatran 150 mg twice daily therapy was superior to warfarin and 110 mg twice daily was noninferior to warfarin in the prevention of stroke for nonvalvular AF. Rates of major hemorrhage were similar to warfarin at 150 mg dosing and

lower at 110 mg dose. Additionally, the annual rate of ICH was lower with dabigatran (0.10% for 150 mg; 0.12% for 110 mg) versus warfarin (0.38%).[8] Rivaroxaban, apixaban, and edoxaban are all factor Xa inhibitors also approved for the prevention of stroke in nonvalvular AF. Large-scale, randomized, controlled studies have also shown a significant decrease in the risk of ICH with the NOACs compared with warfarin.[9–11] A recent metaanalysis of these studies concluded that NOACs in combination with low dose-aspirin may be safer and more effective than warfarin in the prevention of stroke and vascular death and also have a lower incidence of ICH.[12]

Some studies have found that up to 37% of patients with ICH have concurrent AF.[13] Therefore, after determination of whether a patient is at risk for thromboembolism, this risk can then be weighed against scoring systems, which have been used to quantify the annual risk of hemorrhage. Various systems include $HEMORR_2HAGES$,[14] ATRIA,[15] ORBIT,[16] and HAS-BLED.[17] The HAS-BLED system (hypertension, abnormal renal/liver function [1 point for each], history of stroke, bleeding history or predisposition, labile International Normalized Ratio, elderly [age > 65 years], drug/alcohol use [1 point for each]) has demonstrated significant value in ability to predict ICH compared with the other models in patients taking both warfarin and NOACs.[18,19] It has also been useful in risk stratification of recurrence of ICH.[20]

Mechanical Heart Valves

Anticoagulation is recommended in all patients with mechanical heart valves (MHV), owing to their highly thrombogenic nature. Mechanical heart valves require warfarin therapy, and NOACs are not currently used for this indication. The annual risk of thromboembolism has been shown to be decreased from 22.0% to 2.2% in those with mechanical mitral valves and from 12.0% to 1.1% in those with mechanical aortic valves using anticoagulation.[21] A goal International Normalized Ratio of 2.5 to 3.0 is recommended in those with aortic valves and a goal of 3.0 is recommended in those with mitral valve. A daily dose of aspirin of 75 to 100 mg is recommended in these patients as well.[22]

Reinitiation of Anticoagulation in the Setting of Structural Disease After Neurosurgery

After a patient undergoes a neurosurgical procedure or suffers ICH secondary to anticoagulation, one of the most pressing issues regards reinitiation of therapy. The literature is lacking regarding this subject and practices vary by practitioner. The literature regarding the reinitiation of therapy after ICH is more robust, and neurosurgeons may be able to extrapolate the data and apply them to postoperative patients. A survey of neurosurgeons regarding reinitiation of therapy after ICH showed that 47% experienced the issue at least once weekly. The most common restart time was 1 month (43.5%) and most (59.4%) indicated that decisions were made based on own intuition or past experiences.[23]

Reinstitution of these medications has been shown to be necessary and safe. A metaanalysis investigated outcomes after the reinitiation of warfarin and antiplatelet agents after ICH in patients with AF. These patients had a median CHADS$_2$ score of 2. Treatment with warfarin was associated with a decrease of ischemic stroke of 45% to 47% compared with no anticoagulation or antiplatelet therapy only, similar to patients without history of ICH. More important, there was no increase in the risk for recurrence of ICH after resumption of warfarin.[24] These results have recently been confirmed in a large, prospective cohort as well.[25] A population-based, Danish nationwide study examined the outcomes after first-time ICH. Of 6369 patients, 2978 (47%) had an indication for anticoagulant or antiplatelet therapy at the time of follow-up. In these patients, the postdischarge use of antithrombotic therapy was associated with a lower risk of death and thromboembolic events, without an increase in the incidence of major bleeding, including repeat ICH.[26] None of these studies provide any insight as to the timing of the reinitiation of therapy, however.

A separate metaanalysis, focused on outcomes after reinitiation of warfarin after ICH in patients with MHV, found an overall recurrence rate of 13%, with a valve thrombosis rate of 7% and stroke rate of 12%. A trend toward lower ICH recurrence was observed with delayed reinitiation. Analysis suggested 4 to 7 days after stabilization of ICH as an ideal time for restarting warfarin.[27] A recent large, German cohort study of ICH in the setting of MHV showed that the reinitiation of warfarin was associated with significant hemorrhage risk (>3.5% per day) until 2 weeks after ICH. This risk was significantly higher than the rate of thromboembolic complications (0.6% per day) during the same time period. These authors advocated that reinitiation of anticoagulation in patients at very high risk of complications (such as those also with AF) at 6 days after ICH was acceptable. The authors were unwilling to agree with recommendations of the previous metaanalysis to restart anticoagulation at an early timepoint based on calculations of a number needed to harm of 31 patients anticoagulated per day to experience a hemorrhagic complication versus a number needed to harm of 256 per day to experience a thromboembolic complication.[28]

Several studies have investigated the association between chronic subdural hematoma and anticoagulation. A metaanalysis of the results revealed a lack of good evidence regarding this clinical scenario. Reinitiation of anticoagulants, but not antiplatelets, may lead to recurrence of the hematoma; however, some studies have suggested that resumption at 72 hours after evacuation may be safe, because thrombotic complications peaked at that time.[29] Another study of patients with MHV and chronic subdural hematoma demonstrated that anticoagulation could safely be held for 3 weeks without complication.[30] Clearly, the data are mixed and more are needed to make a safe conclusion regarding the reinitiation of these medications in patients with this condition. Each patient must be treated on an individualized basis, with assistance of the risk scales previously mentioned.[31]

MANAGEMENT OF ANTIPLATELETS IN PATIENTS WITH NEUROENDOVASCULAR DEVICES

Over the last 20 years, the endovascular treatment of both unruptured and ruptured aneurysms has significantly evolved, including both the use of balloon and stent-assisted coil placement as well as flow diversion devices.[32] Wide-necked aneurysms have been a focus of these devices; traditionally, the placement of coils within these aneurysms has a very high risk of coil protrusion into the parent vessel, potentially leading to thromboembolism. Stents have been developed to assist with the placement of coils into these aneurysms and have been successful in the elective treatment of aneurysms.[33]

A newer development in the treatment of intracranial aneurysms has been the use of flow diverter devices. These are self-expanding stents with 30% to 35% metal surface area that function by redirecting blood flow past the aneurysm, followed by stagnation of blood, clot formation, remodeling, and eventual endothelial growth across the device. The Pipeline Embolization Device (Medtronic, Minneapolis, MN) is the model currently approved for use in the United States for the treatment of large and giant aneurysms of the internal carotid artery from the petrous segment to the superior hypophyseal segment.[34] Its use has expanded significantly off-label for treatment of a variety of other intracranial aneurysms.[35] Several large studies have demonstrated the effectiveness of flow diversion, including Pipeline for the Intracranial Treatment of Aneurysms (PITA), which showed an aneurysm occlusion rate of 93% at 6 months,[36] and Pipeline for Uncoilable or Failed Aneurysms (PUFS),[37] which showed 73% occlusion at 180 days. The 3-year and 5-year PUFS follow-up have shown 93.4% and 95.2% occlusion rates, respectively.[38]

Placement of devices such as these, as well as carotid artery stents, necessitate the use of dual antiplatelet therapy (DAPT) to prevent thromboembolism and in-device stenosis. However, practitioners need to practice caution, because patients may be hyporesponders or hyperresponders to these medications, potentially causing significant complications. A recent metaanalysis of the flow diverter literature revealed overall rates complications to be 9.9% (6.6% thrombotic, 3% hemorrhagic, 0.3% in-pipeline stenosis).[39]

Typically, patients are pretreated 5 to 7 days before the procedure with both aspirin 325 mg daily and clopidogrel 75 mg/d, although significant variation exists.[39] Before intervention, platelet inhibition can be readily assessed with blood tests such as the VerifyNow-Aspirin and VerifyNow-P2Y12 assays. Both tests produce results that correlate well with results of the more costly and difficult to perform, but gold standard test, light transmittance aggregometry. Aspirin inhibits cyclooxygenase 1, preventing the formation of thromboxane A2, a platelet aggregating prostanoid. VerifyNow tests for failure of aspirin to inhibit thromboxane A2 formation. Platelet inhibition with aspirin is defined as less than 550 aspirin response units. Studies have shown aspirin resistance in up to 26% of the population, with a suggestion that patients on higher doses may have less resistance than on lower doses.[40] Aspirin resistance has also been linked to not taking an angiotensin-converting enzyme inhibitor or angiotensin receptor blocker.[41]

Clopidogrel is a prodrug that requires metabolism to be activated, and functions by binding to the P2Y12 ADP receptor on platelet membranes. The VerifyNow-P2Y12 assay measures the effects of clopidogrel or other P2Y12 inhibitors on the receptor.[40] Appropriate platelet inhibition as assessed with the P2Y12 assay is usually between 60 and 240 platelet response units, with ideal inhibition between 70 and 150 units.[42] Variability in responsiveness to clopidogrel dosing is associated with metabolism of the prodrug owing to cytochrome P450 variants.[43] Resistance rates vary from 21% to 53% in the population.[3] Other factors implicated in resistance include age greater than 55 years, female sex, diabetes, and the use of proton pump inhibitors.[44] Inversely,

smoking can enhance clopidogrel-mediated platelet inhibition.[45]

Careful tailoring of medication regimen is necessary when resistance or hyperresponsiveness is observed. If feasible, procedure delay may be necessary for proper adjustment. In hyperresponsiveness, a decrease from daily dosing to every other day or every third day may be effective. In cases of resistance, dose escalation is 1 option.[46] However, an alternative is to use a newer generation P2Y12 inhibitor, such as prasugrel or ticagrelor, as demonstrated by practitioner preferences.[47] These methods have been shown to be effective, safe alternatives in the setting of neuroendovascular devices. Prasugrel requires less metabolism than clopidogrel and provides a more rapid and consistent inhibition of platelets even in the setting of factors that can affect clopidogrel, such as older age, diabetes, or smoking, as mentioned. It may even lead to a decrease in thromboembolic complications without an increase in hemorrhagic events.[48,49] One study, however, did show an increase in hemorrhagic events using aspirin/prasugrel DAPT, although this was nonsignificant if excluding 1 case involving basilar artery perforation.[50] The loading dose for prasugrel is 60 mg, with a maintenance dose of 10 mg/d.[3] Aspirin/ticagrelor DAPT use with both flow diverter and stent coil cases has shown lower rates of ischemia and similar rates of hemorrhage to those reported previously for aspirin/clopidogrel DAPT.[51] The loading dose for ticagrelor is 180 mg and platelet inhibition achieved in 1 hour (compared with 4–6 hours for 600 mg loading dose of clopidogrel) with a maintenance dose of 90 mg twice daily. Recovery of platelet function after last dose is also faster than with clopidogrel and may be more desirable should emergency situations arise.[52] It must be noted that a US Food and Drug Administration black box warning exists for aspirin/ticagrelor DAPT that aspirin doses of greater than 100 mg/d may reduce the effectiveness of this therapy.[53]

VENOUS THROMBOEMBOLISM IN NEUROSURGICAL PATIENTS

A comprehensive review of the incidence, pathophysiology, diagnosis and prophylaxis against developing VTE has been presented in this series by Shaikhouni and Lonser. We, therefore, focus on its treatment.

Treatment of Venous Thromboembolism

The standard care for treatment of above-the-knee DVT and PE is therapeutic anticoagulation for at least 3 to 6 months after diagnosis. Initial treatment is usually with unfractionated heparin or low-molecular-weight heparin, with transition to oral anticoagulation or continued low-molecular-weight heparin injections in most instances.[54] One small, retrospective study is available concerning outcomes of therapeutic anticoagulation after craniotomy. Forty-two patients with postoperative DVT or PE were diagnosed at a median of 5 days postoperatively. They were treated with therapeutic unfractionated heparin or low-molecular-weight heparin and were fully anticoagulated at a median of 12 days postoperatively. No patients experienced deterioration as evidenced by no change in clinical status or no new hemorrhage on computed tomography scanning of the head.[55] A separate, large, registry-based study of patients with symptomatic, confirmed VTE performed a subanalysis on the natural history of postoperative VTE in both cranial and spinal neurosurgical patients. In the study, 0.96% developed symptomatic VTE within 60 days after surgery, of which the 2 largest subgroups included patients who underwent surgery for malignancy (36%) and those for ICH (15%). Of the patients diagnosed with VTE, 89% underwent initial VTE therapy with low-molecular-weight heparin. Findings demonstrated that, after initiation of therapy, PE is the most fatal complication during the first week (despite therapy) and that, after the first week, the main complication was bleeding.[56]

Inferior Vena Cava Filter Placement

There are currently 2 indications for inferior vena cava (IVC) filter placement: patients with VTE and a contraindication for therapeutic anticoagulation, and patients with recurrent PE despite anticoagulation.[57] It is suggested that IVC filters are strongly considered in patients with acute VTE with contradiction for anticoagulation.[54] There has been recent interest in the use of preoperative IVC filter placement. Most studies have focused on this strategy in the setting of complex spinal surgery, and there seems to be a benefit. One such study found that preoperative IVC filter placement in high-risk patients undergoing complex spine surgery had decreased rates of postoperative PE from 12% to 0% compared with matched control cohorts.[58] Another similar study found decreased incidence of symptomatic postoperative PE from 4.2% to 1.5%.[59] Patients with spinal metastases were also found to have a high rate (9.48%) of preoperative DVT. Nonambulatory patients had a 4-fold increase in DVT incidence over ambulatory patients. All of the patients with DVT underwent preoperative IVC filter placement, and of these patients, only 1 developed a postoperative PE.[60]

INTRATHECAL ACCESS IN PATIENTS ON ANTIPLATELET OR ANTICOAGULATION THERAPY
External Ventricular Drain

External ventricular drain (EVD) placement can be a life-saving procedure for both drainage of cerebral spinal fluid and monitoring of intracranial pressure in the setting of hydrocephalus caused by a variety of neurosurgical conditions. It is a relatively safe procedure, as a recent study showed overall low risk of EVD-related hemorrhage, with an overall occurrence of 7% and a rate of significant hemorrhage of 0.8%.[61] Given the new era of endovascular treatment of aneurysms, patients who present with subarachnoid hemorrhage and hydrocephalus presents a new problem for patients who require EVD placement as more stent coil and flow diverter procedures (with attendant DAPT administration) are being done in the setting of subarachnoid hemorrhage.[62,63] Intravenous heparin administration during therapy is necessary to prevent thromboembolism, with possible continuation of an anticoagulant afterward in the instance of parent vessel thrombus or coil migration.

Several studies have investigated the safety of placement of EVD before endovascular treatment of ruptured aneurysm. Hoh and colleagues[64] showed that heparinization for coiling is safe even after EVD placement within 24 hours. Gard and colleagues[65] further elucidated this finding, showing heparinization to be safe 4 hours after EVD placement, with a tract hemorrhage rate of 6.9%. Two additional studies showed no significant increase in periprocedural EVD and ICP monitor-related hemorrhage.[66,67]

Several other findings contradict these studies, however. In a small, retrospective study, Kung and colleagues[68] found that rates of radiographic and symptomatic hemorrhage were significantly higher in those who underwent stent-assisted coiling with DAPT (32% and 8%) than those that did not have stent-assisted coiling (14.7% and 0.9%). Two additional studies demonstrated that EVD-related hemorrhage is significantly increased in patients who underwent endovascular therapy requiring anticoagulation for aneurysm treatment versus those who received no anticoagulation (coiling or clipping)[69] or versus those who underwent clipping alone.[70] Given these conflicting reports, the safest method of EVD placement in the setting of subarachnoid hemorrhage seems to be placement as soon as possible, before any intervention.

Lumbar Puncture and Lumbar Drain Placement

Lumbar puncture and lumbar drain placement are common procedures used for drainage and/or analysis of cerebrospinal fluid that can be performed by neurosurgeons. However, the literature is lacking regarding guidance on safety of performing these procedures on patients taking anticoagulant and antiplatelet medications. Most data on the subject come from the emergency medicine literature or the anesthesia literature regarding epidural or spinal anesthesia. These data can likely be applied to these procedures. The incidence of spinal epidural hematoma has been estimated at less than 1 in 150,000 epidural and less than 1 in 220,000 spinal anesthetics.[71] A comprehensive review on the topic demonstrates that performing a lumbar puncture or epidural/spinal anesthesia on a patient taking aspirin has a 24.4% rate of minor hemorrhagic complications without evidence of major hemorrhage.[72] The risk of complication associated with discontinuing aspirin has been shown to be 10.2%.[73] Therefore, this procedure may be considered without stopping aspirin therapy.

Patients may also be taking P2Y12 inhibitors such as clopidogrel, prasugrel, or ticagrelor. Stoppage of these is recommended at least 7 days before a planned procedure. There is disagreement between societies as to when to restart these medications, but it has been suggested that they may be safely restarted at 24 hours after neuraxial injection.[74] In those patients on therapeutic heparin, it is recommended to stop the infusion and wait at least 4 hours, given that the half-life of intravenous heparin is 30 to 150 minutes, or until the partial thromboplastin is in the normal range.[75]

Patients on chronic anticoagulation present a more complex challenge. We do not recommend lumbar puncture or lumbar drain in anticoagulated patients. In an emergency setting, treatment with prothrombin complex concentrate as well as vitamin K has been shown to be effective and safe, with a low complication rate.[76] In nonemergent settings, it is recommended to wait at least 5 days after cessation of therapy to perform the procedure. In higher risk patients, it is reasonable to bridge from warfarin to either low-molecular-weight heparin and then perform a lumbar puncture at least 12 hours after last dose or give unfractionated heparin in patients with renal disease and then perform lumbar puncture at least 6 hours after the last dose. Heparin may safely be restarted 1 hour after the procedure.[72]

NOACs present a different problem, because each of them are metabolized in a drug-specific manner and have variable half-lives that can be prolonged in patients with renal dysfunction. It is recommended to wait for a period of 5 half-lives before a procedure, meaning stoppage at least 3 days before a procedure in those with a

creatinine clearance of greater than 50 mL/min and 4 to 5 days in those with a creatinine clearance of less than 50 mL/min.[74]

It is recommended that the same guidelines apply to neuraxial injection, catheter placement, and catheter removal. Guidelines on the reinitiation of medications either after lumbar puncture or removal of lumbar drain catheter vary for each medication, but these can likely be resumed at a minimum of 24 to 48 hours in most patients. Of course, management of each patient should follow guidelines as discussed elsewhere in this article.

SUMMARY

Neurosurgeons clearly very commonly encounter patients who require anticoagulation and antiplatelet therapy. Knowledge of when to restart these medications after procedures as well as how to manage them periprocedurally to balance the risks of thromboembolism and hemorrhage is complex. Some literature assists in this endeavor, aiding in risk stratification; however, much remains unclear. Platelet function testing is a well-documented method in guiding antiplatelet therapy for patients with neuroendovascular devices, but it may be difficult to interpret results and safely alter medication regimens to balance a patient's safety and risks. Patients necessitate individual treatment algorithms and should be involved in the process. As the population ages, this task will only become more common, and likely more difficult, but with basic knowledge of the landscape, neurosurgeons can better serve their patients and optimize outcomes.

REFERENCES

1. Barnes GD, Lucas E, Alexander GC, et al. National trends in ambulatory oral anticoagulant use. Am J Med 2015;128(12):1300–5.e2.
2. Gu Q, Dillon CF, Eberhardt MS, et al. Preventive aspirin and other antiplatelet medication use among U.S. Adults aged >/= 40 years: data from the National Health and nutrition examination survey, 2011-2012. Public Health Rep 2015;130(6):643–54.
3. Kim KS, Fraser JF, Grupke S, et al. Management of antiplatelet therapy in patients undergoing neuroendovascular procedures. J Neurosurg 2017;1–16.
4. Colilla S, Crow A, Petkun W, et al. Estimates of current and future incidence and prevalence of atrial fibrillation in the U.S. adult population. Am J Cardiol 2013;112(8):1142–7.
5. January CT, Wann LS, Alpert JS, et al. 2014 AHA/ACC/HRS guideline for the management of patients with atrial fibrillation: a report of the American College of Cardiology/American Heart Association

Task Force on practice guidelines and the Heart Rhythm Society. Circulation 2014;130(23):e199–267.

6. Kirchhof P, Benussi S, Kotecha D, et al. 2016 ESC Guidelines for the management of atrial fibrillation developed in collaboration with EACTS. Eur Heart J 2016;37(38):2893–962.

7. Risk factors for stroke and efficacy of antithrombotic therapy in atrial fibrillation. Analysis of pooled data from five randomized controlled trials. Arch Intern Med 1994;154(13):1449–57.

8. Manjila S, Masri T, Shams T, et al. Evidence-based review of primary and secondary ischemic stroke prevention in adults: a neurosurgical perspective. Neurosurg Focus 2011;30(6):E1.

9. Patel MR, Mahaffey KW, Garg J, et al. Rivaroxaban versus warfarin in nonvalvular atrial fibrillation. N Engl J Med 2011;365(10):883–91.

10. Granger CB, Alexander JH, McMurray JJ, et al. Apixaban versus warfarin in patients with atrial fibrillation. N Engl J Med 2011;365(11):981–92.

11. Giugliano RP, Ruff CT, Braunwald E, et al. Edoxaban versus warfarin in patients with atrial fibrillation. N Engl J Med 2013;369(22):2093–104.

12. Bennaghmouch N, de Veer AJWM, Bode K, et al. Efficacy and safety of the use of non-vitamin k antagonist oral anticoagulants in patients with nonvalvular atrial fibrillation and concomitant aspirin therapy: a meta-analysis of randomized trials. Circulation 2018;137(11):1117–29.

13. Horstmann S, Rizos T, Jenetzky E, et al. Prevalence of atrial fibrillation in intracerebral hemorrhage. Eur J Neurol 2014;21(4):570–6.

14. Gage BF, Yan Y, Milligan PE, et al. Clinical classification schemes for predicting hemorrhage: results from the National Registry of Atrial Fibrillation (NRAF). Am Heart J 2006;151(3):713–9.

15. Fang MC, Go AS, Chang Y, et al. A new risk scheme to predict warfarin-associated hemorrhage: the ATRIA (Anticoagulation and Risk Factors in Atrial Fibrillation) study. J Am Coll Cardiol 2011;58(4):395–401.

16. O'Brien EC, Simon DN, Thomas LE, et al. The ORBIT bleeding score: a simple bedside score to assess bleeding risk in atrial fibrillation. Eur Heart J 2015; 36(46):3258–64.

17. Pisters R, Lane DA, Nieuwlaat R, et al. A novel user-friendly score (HAS-BLED) to assess 1-year risk of major bleeding in patients with atrial fibrillation: the Euro Heart Survey. Chest 2010;138(5):1093–100.

18. Senoo K, Proietti M, Lane DA, et al. Evaluation of the HAS-BLED, ATRIA, and ORBIT bleeding risk scores in patients with atrial fibrillation taking warfarin. Am J Med 2016;129(6):600–7.

19. Apostolakis S, Lane DA, Guo Y, et al. Performance of the HEMORR 2 HAGES, ATRIA, and HAS-BLED bleeding risk-prediction scores in nonwarfarin anti-coagulated atrial fibrillation patients. J Am Coll Cardiol 2013;61(3):386–7.

20. Chan KH, Ka-Kit Leung G, Lau KK, et al. Predictive value of the HAS-BLED score for the risk of recurrent intracranial hemorrhage after first spontaneous intracranial hemorrhage. World Neurosurg 2014;82(1–2): e219–23.

21. Baudet EM, Puel V, McBride JT, et al. Long-term results of valve replacement with the St. Jude Medical prosthesis. J Thorac Cardiovasc Surg 1995;109(5): 858–70.

22. Nishimura RA, Otto CM, Bonow RO, et al. 2017 AHA/ACC focused update of the 2014 AHA/ACC guideline for the management of patients with valvular heart disease: a report of the American College of Cardiology/American Heart Association Task Force on Clinical Practice Guidelines. Circulation 2017; 135(25):e1159–95.

23. Hawryluk GW, Furlan JC, Austin JW, et al. Survey of neurosurgical management of central nervous system hemorrhage in patients receiving anticoagulation therapy: current practice is highly variable and may be suboptimal. World Neurosurg 2011; 76(3–4):299–303.

24. Korompoki E, Filippidis FT, Nielsen PB, et al. Long-term antithrombotic treatment in intracranial hemorrhage survivors with atrial fibrillation. Neurology 2017;89(7):687–96.

25. Poli L, Grassi M, Zedde M, et al. Anticoagulants resumption after warfarin-related intracerebral haemorrhage: the multicenter study on cerebral hemorrhage in Italy (MUCH-Italy). Thromb Haemost 2018; 118(3):572–80.

26. Ottosen TP, Grijota M, Hansen ML, et al. Use of antithrombotic therapy and long-term clinical outcome among patients surviving intracerebral hemorrhage. Stroke 2016;47(7):1837–43.

27. AlKherayf F, Xu Y, Gandara E, et al. Timing of vitamin K antagonist re-initiation following intracranial hemorrhage in mechanical heart valves: systematic review and meta-analysis. Thromb Res 2016;144: 152–7.

28. Kuramatsu JB, Sembill JA, Gerner ST, et al. Management of therapeutic anticoagulation in patients with intracerebral haemorrhage and mechanical heart valves. Eur Heart J 2018;39(19):1709–23.

29. Nathan S, Goodarzi Z, Jette N, et al. Anticoagulant and antiplatelet use in seniors with chronic subdural hematoma: systematic review. Neurology 2017; 88(20):1889–93.

30. Amin AG, Ng J, Hsu W, et al. Postoperative anticoagulation in patients with mechanical heart valves following surgical treatment of subdural hematomas. Neurocrit Care 2013;19(1):90–4.

31. Guha D, Macdonald RL. Perioperative management of anticoagulation. Neurosurg Clin N Am 2017;28(2): 287–95.

32. Rajah G, Narayanan S, Rangel-Castilla L. Update on flow diverters for the endovascular management

of cerebral aneurysms. Neurosurg Focus 2017; 42(6):E2.

33. Benitez RP, Silva MT, Klem J, et al. Endovascular occlusion of wide-necked aneurysms with a new intracranial microstent (Neuroform) and detachable coils. Neurosurgery 2004;54(6):1359–67 [discussion: 1368].

34. Al-Mufti F, Amuluru K, Gandhi CD, et al. Flow diversion for intracranial aneurysm management: a new standard of care. Neurotherapeutics 2016;13(3): 582–9.

35. Patel PD, Chalouhi N, Atallah E, et al. Off-label uses of the Pipeline embolization device: a review of the literature. Neurosurg Focus 2017;42(6):E4.

36. Nelson PK, Lylyk P, Szikora I, et al. The pipeline embolization device for the intracranial treatment of aneurysms trial. AJNR Am J Neuroradiol 2011; 32(1):34–40.

37. Sahlein DH, Fouladvand M, Becske T, et al. Neuroophthalmological outcomes associated with use of the pipeline embolization device: analysis of the PUFS trial results. J Neurosurg 2015;123(4): 897–905.

38. Becske T, Brinjikji W, Potts MB, et al. Long-term clinical and angiographic outcomes following pipeline embolization device treatment of complex internal carotid artery aneurysms: five-year results of the pipeline for uncoilable or failed aneurysms trial. Neurosurgery 2017;80(1):40–8.

39. Texakalidis P, Bekelis K, Atallah E, et al. Flow diversion with the pipeline embolization device for patients with intracranial aneurysms and antiplatelet therapy: a systematic literature review. Clin Neurol Neurosurg 2017;161:78–87.

40. Oxley TJ, Dowling RJ, Mitchell PJ, et al. Antiplatelet resistance and thromboembolic complications in neurointerventional procedures. Front Neurol 2011; 2:83.

41. Reavey-Cantwell JF, Fox WC, Reichwage BD, et al. Factors associated with aspirin resistance in patients premedicated with aspirin and clopidogrel for endovascular neurosurgery. Neurosurgery 2009;64(5):890–5 [discussion: 895–6].

42. Daou B, Starke RM, Chalouhi N, et al. P2Y12 reaction units: effect on hemorrhagic and thromboembolic complications in patients with cerebral aneurysms treated with the pipeline embolization device. Neurosurgery 2016;78(1):27–33.

43. Mega JL, Close SL, Wiviott SD, et al. Cytochrome p-450 polymorphisms and response to clopidogrel. N Engl J Med 2009;360(4):354–62.

44. Prabhakaran S, Wells KR, Lee VH, et al. Prevalence and risk factors for aspirin and clopidogrel resistance in cerebrovascular stenting. AJNR Am J Neuroradiol 2008;29(2):281–5.

45. Gremmel T, Steiner S, Seidinger D, et al. Smoking promotes clopidogrel-mediated platelet inhibition in patients receiving dual antiplatelet therapy. Thromb Res 2009;124(5):588–91.

46. Roberts DI, Nawarskas JJ. Treatment options for patients with poor clopidogrel response. Cardiol Rev 2013;21(6):309–17.

47. Gupta R, Moore JM, Griessenauer CJ, et al. Assessment of dual-antiplatelet regimen for pipeline embolization device placement: a survey of major academic neurovascular centers in the United States. World Neurosurg 2016;96:285–92.

48. Choi HH, Lee JJ, Cho YD, et al. Antiplatelet premedication for stent-assisted coil embolization of intracranial aneurysms: low-dose prasugrel vs clopidogrel. Neurosurgery 2017. [Epub ahead of print].

49. Sedat J, Chau Y, Gaudart J, et al. Prasugrel versus clopidogrel in stent-assisted coil embolization of unruptured intracranial aneurysms. Interv Neuroradiol 2017;23(1):52–9.

50. Akbari SH, Reynolds MR, Kadkhodayan Y, et al. Hemorrhagic complications after prasugrel (Effient) therapy for vascular neurointerventional procedures. J Neurointerv Surg 2013;5(4):337–43.

51. Narata AP, Amelot A, Bibi R, et al. Dual antiplatelet therapy combining aspirin and ticagrelor for intracranial stenting procedures: a retrospective single center study of 154 consecutive patients with unruptured aneurysms. Neurosurgery 2018. [Epub ahead of print].

52. Gurbel PA, Bliden KP, Butler K, et al. Randomized double-blind assessment of the ONSET and OFFSET of the antiplatelet effects of ticagrelor versus clopidogrel in patients with stable coronary artery disease: the ONSET/OFFSET study. Circulation 2009; 120(25):2577–85.

53. Serebruany VL. Ticagrelor FDA approval issues revisited. Cardiology 2012;122(3):144–7.

54. Streiff MB, Agnelli G, Connors JM, et al. Guidance for the treatment of deep vein thrombosis and pulmonary embolism. J Thromb Thrombolysis 2016; 41(1):32–67.

55. Scheller C, Rachinger J, Strauss C, et al. Therapeutic anticoagulation after craniotomies: is the risk for secondary hemorrhage overestimated? J Neurol Surg A Cent Eur Neurosurg 2014;75(1):2–6.

56. Cote LP, Greenberg S, Caprini JA, et al. Outcomes in neurosurgical patients who develop venous thromboembolism: a review of the RIETE registry. Clin Appl Thromb Hemost 2014;20(8):772–8.

57. Wehrenberg-Klee E, Stavropoulos SW. Inferior vena cava filters for primary prophylaxis: when are they indicated? Semin Intervent Radiol 2012; 29(1):29–35.

58. Rosner MK, Kuklo TR, Tawk R, et al. Prophylactic placement of an inferior vena cava filter in high-risk patients undergoing spinal reconstruction. Neurosurg Focus 2004;17(4):E6.

59. Ozturk C, Ganiyusufoglu K, Alanay A, et al. Efficacy of prophylactic placement of inferior vena cava filter in patients undergoing spinal surgery. Spine (Phila Pa 1976) 2010;35(20):1893–6.

60. Zacharia BE, Kahn S, Bander ED, et al. Incidence and risk factors for preoperative deep venous thrombosis in 314 consecutive patients undergoing surgery for spinal metastasis. J Neurosurg Spine 2017;27(2):189–97.

61. Bauer DF, Razdan SN, Bartolucci AA, et al. Meta-analysis of hemorrhagic complications from ventriculostomy placement by neurosurgeons. Neurosurgery 2011;69(2):255–60.

62. Amenta PS, Dalyai RT, Kung D, et al. Stent-assisted coiling of wide-necked aneurysms in the setting of acute subarachnoid hemorrhage: experience in 65 patients. Neurosurgery 2012;70(6):1415–29 [discussion: 1429].

63. Natarajan SK, Shallwani H, Fennell VS, et al. Flow diversion after aneurysmal subarachnoid hemorrhage. Neurosurg Clin N Am 2017;28(3):375–88.

64. Hoh BL, Nogueira RG, Ledezma CJ, et al. Safety of heparinization for cerebral aneurysm coiling soon after external ventriculostomy drain placement. Neurosurgery 2005;57(5):845–9 [discussion: 845–9].

65. Gard AP, Sayles BD, Robbins JW, et al. Hemorrhage rate after external ventricular drain placement in subarachnoid hemorrhage: time to heparin administration. Neurocrit Care 2017;27(3):350–5.

66. Leschke JM, Lozen A, Kaushal M, et al. Hemorrhagic complications associated with ventriculostomy in patients undergoing endovascular treatment for intracranial aneurysms: a single-center experience. Neurocrit Care 2017;27(1):11–6.

67. Scholz C, Hubbe U, Deininger M, et al. Hemorrhage rates of external ventricular drain (EVD), intracranial pressure gauge (ICP) or combined EVD and ICP gauge placement within 48 h of endovascular coil embolization of cerebral aneurysms. Clin Neurol Neurosurg 2013;115(8):1399–402.

68. Kung DK, Policeni BA, Capuano AW, et al. Risk of ventriculostomy-related hemorrhage in patients with acutely ruptured aneurysms treated using stent-assisted coiling. J Neurosurg 2011;114(4):1021–7.

69. Bruder M, Schuss P, Konczalla J, et al. Ventriculostomy-related hemorrhage after treatment of acutely ruptured aneurysms: the influence of anticoagulation and antiplatelet treatment. World Neurosurg 2015;84(6):1653–9.

70. Scheller C, Strauss C, Prell J, et al. Increased rate of ventriculostomy-related hemorrhage following endovascular treatment of ruptured aneurysms compared to clipping. Acta Neurochir (Wien) 2018;160(3):545–50.

71. Horlocker TT, Wedel DJ. Neurologic complications of spinal and epidural anesthesia. Reg Anesth Pain Med 2000;25(1):83–98.

72. Domingues R, Bruniera G, Brunale F, et al. Lumbar puncture in patients using anticoagulants and antiplatelet agents. Arq Neuropsiquiatr 2016;74(8):679–86.

73. Hillemacher T, Bleich S, Wiltfang J, et al. Should aspirin be discontinued for diagnostic lumbar puncture? J Am Geriatr Soc 2006;54(1):181–2.

74. Benzon HT, Avram MJ, Green D, et al. New oral anticoagulants and regional anaesthesia. Br J Anaesth 2013;111(Suppl 1):i96–113.

75. Liu SS, Mulroy MF. Neuraxial anesthesia and analgesia in the presence of standard heparin. Reg Anesth Pain Med 1998;23(6 Suppl 2):157–63.

76. Lalble M, Beynon C, Sander P, et al. Treatment with prothrombin complex concentrate to enable emergency lumbar puncture in patients receiving vitamin K antagonists. Ann Emerg Med 2016;68(3):340–4.

Section IV: Treatment of Thrombosis in the Neurosurgical Patient

Management of Venous Sinus Thrombosis

Nicholas Sader, MD[a], Madeleine de Lotbinière-Bassett, MD[a], Michael K. Tso, MD[a], Mark Hamilton, MDCM, FRCSC[b],*

KEYWORDS

- Cerebral thrombosis • Sinus thrombosis • Cerebral venous sinus thrombosis • Venous stroke
- Anticoagulation • Heparin • Low molecular weight heparin

KEY POINTS

- Cerebral venous sinus thrombosis (CVST) is an uncommon cerebrovascular condition that is more common in middle aged adults and children.
- The signs and symptoms of CVST are highly variable in type and duration, with the most common symptom being headache.
- Imaging with MRI/magnetic resonance venography (MRV) for the diagnosis of CVST, with computed tomography (CT)/CTV (CT venogram) as an alternative is reasonable when MRI is not available.
- First-line treatment is anticoagulation with heparin, even if intracerebral hemorrhage is present.
- Although potentially a fatal disorder, with mortality reported between 8% and 10%, the long-term prognosis is generally positive. Approximately 80% of individuals do not have lasting physical disability from CVST.

INTRODUCTION

Thrombosis of the cerebral veins and sinuses, or cerebral venous sinus thrombosis (CVST), is a rare subtype of cerebrovascular disease representing 0.5% of strokes.[1] This entity was first described over 150 years ago from an autopsy and was believed to have been the cause of death.[2] CVST is seen more frequently in middle aged adults and children, in comparison to arterial strokes that occur more commonly in an older age group. Women are at increased risk of developing CVST because of the hormones associated with the use of oral contraceptives, pregnancy, and the puerperium period.

The signs and symptoms of CVST are often nonspecific and vary in duration and may therefore delay both the diagnosis and treatment. However, increased awareness in the medical community and significant advancements in imaging modalities have resulted in faster diagnosis and therefore improved patient outcomes.

Diagnosis of CVST is typically made using MRI/MRV (MR venogram) or with CT/CTV (CT venogram) as an alternative when MRI is not available. The desired initial treatment is with low molecular weight heparin (LMWH), as opposed to unfractionated heparin (UFH). After the acute stage of CVST, unless there are

Disclosure Statement: The authors have nothing to disclose.
[a] Division of Neurosurgery, Department of Clinical Neurosciences, University of Calgary, Foothills Hospital, 12th Floor, 1403 - 29th Street Northwest, Calgary, Alberta T2N 2T9, Canada; [b] Adult Hydrocephalus Program, Division of Neurosurgery, Department of Clinical Neurosciences, University of Calgary, Adult Hydrocephalus Clinical Research Network, Foothills Hospital, 12th Floor, 1403 - 29th Street Northwest, Calgary, Alberta T2N 2T9, Canada
* Corresponding author.
E-mail address: mghamilton.hydro@gmail.com

Neurosurg Clin N Am 29 (2018) 585–594
https://doi.org/10.1016/j.nec.2018.06.011
1042-3680/18/© 2018 Elsevier Inc. All rights reserved.

neurosurgery.theclinics.com

contraindications, the use of a vitamin K antagonist as an oral anticoagulant (OAC) therapy is currently recommended. Factor Xa inhibitor drugs will likely eventually replace this recommendation.

EPIDEMIOLOGY

CVST is a cerebrovascular disease that is gaining increased detection and earlier treatment because of the development of noninvasive imaging modalities such as MRI and increased awareness in the medical community.[2] The true incidence of CVST is unknown, but was previously estimated to be 5 cases per million population.[1] Historically, incidence was based off autopsy studies that likely underestimated the true value.[2,3] It is generally accepted that the incidence of CVST is higher than previously thought, with recent studies out of the Netherlands and Australia suggesting that the incidence lies between 13.2 and 15.7 cases per million population.[4,5] CVST is also a disease that affects younger individuals, more commonly female as highlighted in the International Study of Cerebral Venous Thrombosis (ISCVT), which included 624 subjects, with a median age of 37 years with 74.5% female patients.[6]

ANATOMY/PATHOPHYSIOLOGY

CVST is described as an evolving disease of prothrombotic and thrombolytic processes that lead to the pathologic initiation and progression of venous thrombosis. The most common venous channels affected are the superior sagittal sinus (72%) and the transverse sinus (70%).[2] The cerebral venous system contains more numerous anastomoses than the cerebral arterial system. A thrombus situated in the venous system can lead to decreased venous drainage, leading to recruitment of collateral vessels. If drainage is insufficient, and the thrombus is situated in a cortical vein, rises in venous capillary pressure may lead to a disruption of the blood-brain barrier, resulting in cerebral edema, ischemia, and possible hemorrhage. Venous strokes are associated with more edema and less necrosis than arterial strokes and are typically associated with a better prognosis.[2] The edema associated with CVST can be of 2 types: cytotoxic or vasogenic. Ischemia leads to intracellular swelling through damage to energy-dependent membrane pumps. Disruption of the blood-brain barrier then results in leakage of blood components into the extracellular space.

If the thrombus is located in the major dural sinuses, intracranial hypertension may occur secondary to increased venous pressure and less significantly from impairment of the arachnoid villi located in the walls of the sagittal sinus. The arachnoid granulations are partially responsible for the absorption of cerebrospinal fluid (CSF) from the subarachnoid space. These 2 mechanisms likely occur simultaneously in most patients.[7]

RISK FACTORS

Several risk factors for thrombus formation have been identified in patients with CVST (**Box 1**). In the International Study on Cerebral Vein and Dural Sinus Thrombosis (ISCVT) trial, 85% of patients had one determined risk factor, and 44% had multiple risk factors.[6] Cerebral and dural thrombosis is three times more common in women than men. This marked discrepancy is thought to be caused by hormonal states that are unique to women, such as pregnancy, the puerperium period, and oral contraceptives.[8,9] The estimated risk of intracranial thrombosis in pregnancy and the puerperium period is 12 cases per 100,000 deliveries, which is only slightly lower than arterial strokes in this same time period.[10]

Neurosurgical procedures may serve as both a treatment and trigger for CVST. A recent retrospective study looked at 2226 patients undergoing a craniotomy for tumor removal found 35 patients (1.5%) went on to develop CVST. The study found that having known CVST risk factors, intraoperative sinus surgery and a semisitting patient positioning during the surgery were all associated with the development of CVST.[11]

CVST risk factors are numerous, and **Table 1** summarizes the most common associations.

CLINICAL FEATURES

The signs and symptoms of CVST are highly variable in both duration and type. **Table 1** outlines the most common presenting symptoms.[6] Headache is by far the most common symptom, occurring in 70% to 75% of patients and typically appearing before any other neurologic symptom.[2] The headache related to CVST may be of sudden onset, often mimicking that of subarachnoid hemorrhage.[12] In certain cases, headache may be the only presenting symptom. Failure to recognize this as a potential symptom of CVST may delay diagnosis and the initiation of treatment, and therefore worsen prognosis.

Seizures occur in approximately 40% of CVST patients, with around 50% of these being of focal onset.[7] The rate of seizure is higher than in arterial strokes.[13]

Four presenting clinical patterns of CVST have been identified[1,2,7]:

Box 1
Risk factors associated with cerebral venous sinus thrombosis

Thrombophilia
Genetic
   Protein C and S deficiency
   Antithrombin deficiency
   Prothrombin G20210A mutation
   Hyperhomocysteinemia
   Factor V Leiden mutation
Acquired
   Pregnancy
   Puerperium
   Nephrotic syndrome
   Antiphospholipid syndrome

Drugs
Oral contraceptives
Hormone replacement therapy
Steroids
Asparaginase

Hematologic disease
Polycythemia
Thrombocythemia
Iron deficiency anemia
Paroxysmal hemoglobinuria

Systemic diseases
Malignancy
Systemic lupus erythematosus
Behcet disease
Rheumatoid arthritis
Thromboangiitis obliterans
Wegener granulomatosis
Inflammatory bowel disease
Sarcoidosis
Thyroid disease

Infection
Ear, sinus, mouth, face, and neck
Meningitis

Mechanical causes
Lumbar puncture
Cranial trauma
Jugular vein catheterization
Neurosurgery procedures

Central nervous system vascular malformations

Dural arteriovenous fistula

AVM

Miscellaneous

Dehydration

Obesity

Data from Refs.[2,7,12]

- Isolated intracranial hypertension- patients usually present with headache, nausea, papilledema and possibly sixth cranial nerve palsy with diplopia
- Focal neurologic deficit or partial seizures-patients have a focal motor and/or sensory deficits
- Subacute diffuse encephalopathy- decreased level of consciousness with no clear focal signs or symptoms
- Painful ophthalmalgia- alludes to cavernous sinus thrombosis with chemosis, proptosis, and ophthalmoplegia caused by affected oculomotor, trochlear, and abducens nerves.

ESTABLISHING A DIAGNOSIS
Laboratory Investigations

The clinical presentation of CVST is highly variable, and therefore the definitive diagnosis relies on further laboratory and imaging investigations (**Fig. 1**). Laboratory investigations are useful in understanding the conditions associated with, or underlying, CVST, but are not diagnostic of

Table 1	
Signs and symptoms of cerebral venous sinus thrombosis	
	Frequency (%)
Headaches	89
Focal motor deficit	41
Seizures	39
Papilledema	28
Aphasia	19
Decreased level of consciousness	14
Diplopia	14
Visual loss	13

From Ferro JM, Canhão P, Stam J, et al. Prognosis of cerebral vein and dural sinus thrombosis: results of the International Study on Cerebral Vein and Dural Sinus Thrombosis (ISCVT). Stroke 2004;35(3):666; with permission.

the disease itself.[13] Initial workup of CVST should involve basic blood work, including a complete blood cell count, chemistry panel, coagulation profile, and urinalysis.[13] D-dimer levels are usually elevated in the acute period of CVST; however, they are not diagnostic of this condition.[1,2] Lumbar puncture should be reserved for specific circumstances, such as in case of suspected central nervous system (CNS) infection.[13] In certain cases the opening pressure, measured during the lumbar puncture procedure, may be useful in determining the intracranial pressure (ICP) and may also serve as therapeutic management by relieving elevated CSF pressure.

Diagnostic Imaging

The next steps in diagnosis of CVST involve neuroimaging, in particular, noncontrast CT head, CTV, MRI head, MRV, and conventional angiography (**Figs. 2** and **3**).[13] Both the American Heart Association (AHA) and the European Academy of Neurology (EAN) guidelines recommend MRI/MRV for the diagnosis of CVST, with CT/CTV as an alternative when MRI is not available.[14–16] In patients who are unstable, or with contraindications to MRI, CTV is sufficient for the identification of CVST.[13] In fact, both the sensitivity and specificity of CT angiography alone for the diagnosis of CVST are 100%.[17]

If present on imaging, certain patterns of intraparenchymal hemorrhage should raise concern for CVST, in particular if the lesion crosses arterial boundaries.[13] If CT imaging within the first hours after symptom onset demonstrate clearly demarcated borders or disproportionate space-occupying lesions, CVST should be high on the differential diagnosis.[13] In approximately one-third of patients with nonhemorrhagic CVST, bilateral parenchymal lesions are present.[13]

Computed tomography

On noncontrast CT, the dense cord sign represents the high density of thrombosis in a sinus or cortical vein.[14] The presence of cerebral infarction

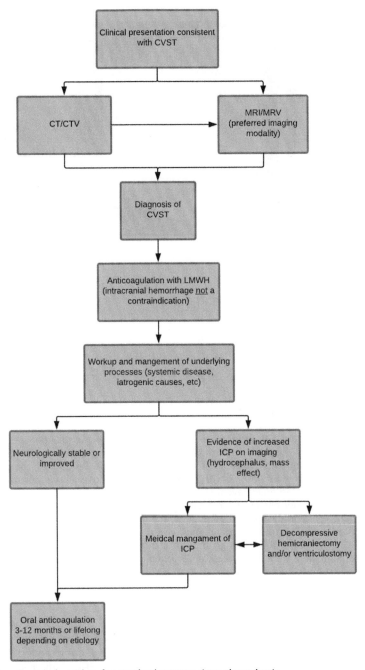

Fig. 1. Diagnosis-treatment algorithm for cerebral venous sinus thrombosis.

outside typical arterial territories, hemorrhage infarct, and bilateral hemorrhages on CT also suggest the presence of CVST.[14] The empty delta sign represents thrombosis in the superior sagittal sinus or the transverse sinus on CTV.[14] The advantages of CT/CTV include the wide and rapid availability of this imaging modality.[14] Limited visualization of cortical and deep CVST, exposure to radiation, and intravenous contrast are potential disadvantages of CT.[13,14] However, 3-dimensional

reconstruction of the CTV can ameliorate the visualization of the affected venous sinus.[14] CTV is generally accepted as a viable alternative to MRI when MRI is either contraindicated or unavailable.[13,14]

MRI

Visualization of the thrombus on T1-weighted images and loss of signal in the venous system on MRV are the most common signs of CVST on

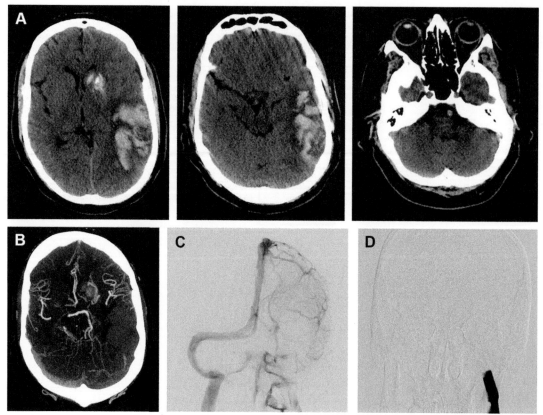

Fig. 2. A 61-year-old man presented with sudden onset of headache, aphasia, right-sided weakness, and a generalized seizure. An unenhanced CT head (*A*) demonstrated a large acute intraparenchymal hemorrhage centered in the left temporoparietal region with 6 mm of left-to-right midline shift. On CTA (*B*), there was nonopacification of the left transverse and sigmoid sinuses, with an intraluminal filling defect demonstrated within the left internal jugular vein. He was started on intravenous heparin and was brought for transvenous thrombolysis. On cerebral angiogram (*C*), an anterior-posterior projection of a left internal carotid artery (ICA) injection revealed occlusion of the left transverse sinus (TS), sigmoid sinus (SS), and internal jugular vein (IJV). The microcatheter was inserted retrograde into the left midtransverse sinus, and a retrievable stent was deployed in the left SS and left IJV. However, this did not improve flow through the left transverse sinus based on the left ICA injection (*D*) showing occlusion. No permanent stent was placed. Unfortunately, the patient after the procedure had increased cerebral swelling and succumbed to his disease.

MRI (see **Fig. 3**D).[14] MRV should be used in combination with MRI, as MRV has several limitations when used in isolation, particularly in cases of thrombosis of a cortical vein or partial sinus occlusion.[13]

The process of blood product degradation can complicate the visualization of CVST on MRI in the acute phases.[14] During the first 5 days after thrombus formation, the increased deoxyhemoglobin content causes the thrombus to appear isointense on T1 images and hypointense on T2 images.[14] The thrombus subsequently becomes hyperintense on both T1- and T2-weighted images during the subacute period, which includes days 5 to 15.[14] The thrombus then becomes homogeneous and hypointense on all imaging sequences after day 15.[14] Use of T2-weighted gradient-recalled echo (GRE) or susceptibility-weighted imaging (SWI) is recommended for visualization of thrombus on MRI, particularly during the acute phase.[13] In MRV, contrast-enhanced imaging is more sensitive for the diagnosis of CVST than time-of-flight imaging.[13]

Digital subtraction angiography
The most accurate method for CVST diagnosis is digital subtraction angiography (DSA) (see **Fig. 2**C, D). However, with the current image quality of CT and MRI scans, DSA is rarely required.[13] DSA is an invasive procedure and carries a small risk of stroke.[13] DSA should be reserved for situations in which other imaging modalities are not

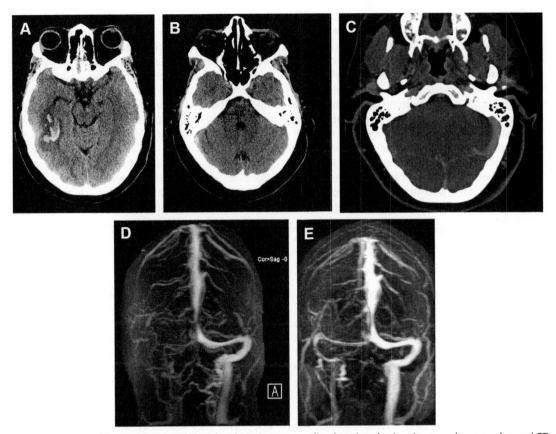

Fig. 3. A 43-year-old woman presented with a first-time generalized tonic-colonic seizure and a nonenhanced CT head (*A*) and demonstrated a moderate sized intraparenchymal hematoma, centered predominantly in the posterosuperior aspect of the right temporal lobe. On CT imaging, a hyperdensity was noted in the distal aspect of the right transverse sinus (*B*). Subsequent CTV and MRV (*C*, *D*) studies confirmed acute right transverse, sigmoid sinus, and internal jugular vein thromboses. The patient was treated with intravenous heparin and subsequently transitioned to warfarin. Follow-up imaging done 1 year later (*E*) demonstrated recanalization of the right transverse and sigmoid sinuses with contrast-enhanced signal seen in the right internal jugular vein.

available, or the diagnosis of CVST remains uncertain or as part of an endovascular treatment strategy.[14]

TREATMENT
Acute General Management

The initial presentation of CVST varies greatly with respect to clinical severity, ranging from headache to increased ICP causing cerebral herniation (see **Fig. 1**).[7] For this reason, initial management should focus on the clinical stabilization of the patient.[7] In the advent of critical increased ICP, treatment may range from medical treatment with intravenous mannitol to decompressive hemicraniectomy.[7] Patients newly diagnosed with CVST should be admitted to the hospital, preferentially to a unit well-versed in the management of intracranial pathology.[7,13] Underlying conditions identified in the initial workup should be addressed.[13] In particular,

dehydration and infection should be appropriately investigated and managed during the acute period.[13]

Patients who present with seizures should be treated with antiepileptic drugs.[13,16] However, the exact duration of treatment is unclear.[13] The use of prophylactic treatment with antiepileptic drugs in CVST is not recommended.[2]

Current guidelines do not include any recommendation for the use of corticosteroids during the treatment of CVST.[18] In fact, in a post hoc analysis of the International Study on Cerebral Vein and Dural Sinus Thrombosis, corticosteroids were found to be detrimental in patients without parenchymal lesions.[18]

Anticoagulation
Heparin The goals of initial treatment for CVST are inhibition of ongoing thrombosis and

recanalization of the thrombosed vessel.[14] The use of heparin for treatment of CVST remained controversial for many decades because of concern regarding the risk of causing or aggravating intracerebral hemorrhage (ICH).[13] In 2011, a meta-analysis of 2 randomized trials including a total of 79 patients demonstrated a nonsignificant difference in favor of therapeutic treatment with heparin.[19] Although this trial did not demonstrate statistical significance, the findings were important clinically, as no new ICH formation occurred in the patients treated with heparin, whereas 2 patients in the control group experienced ICH.[19] In addition, 2 patients in the control group were diagnosed with pulmonary embolism.[19] Current guidelines from the AHA and EAN recommend therapeutic anticoagulation of CVST regardless of the presence of ICH.[15,16]

The current literature suggests that LMWH may be superior to UFH in the treatment of CVST.[13,16] However, no large high-quality randomized trial has confirmed this conclusion.[16,19] LMWH is frequently associated with a decreased risk of thrombotic complications, major bleeding, and death compared with UFH.[20] For these reasons it is recommended that patients be treated with LMWH as opposed to UFH in the context of CVST.[13,16] The use of UFH should be reserved for circumstances in which a contraindication to LMWH exists (eg, renal insufficiency) or when the capacity for fast reversal of anticoagulation is desired (such as in patients who may undergo neurosurgical procedures).[16]

Oral anticoagulation After the acute stage of CVST, unless there are contraindications, the use of a vitamin K antagonist (eg, warfarin) as OAC therapy is recommended.[2,13,16] The international normalized ratio (INR) should be used to target a range between 2.0 and 3.0. If the etiology of CVST is idiopathic or caused by mild thrombophilia, the recommended duration of OAC therapy is 6 to 12 months.[2] In patients with 1 episode of CVST and transient risk factor such as meningitis or trauma, OAC therapy should continue for at least 3 months.[2] Lifelong OAC therapy is recommended in patients with 1 episode of CVST and a severe form of thrombophilia or in patients with 2 or more episodes of CVST.[2]

Factor Xa inhibitors are being used more commonly in general care, and there is some early experience published reporting on their use in patients with CVST.[13,16,21] However, there is no current recommendation to consider the routine use of factor Xa inhibitors drugs during treatment of CVST.[13,16]

Endovascular treatment To date, the evidence supporting the use of endovascular treatment for CVST is limited to case reports and small case series.[19] The endovascular approach to CVST includes both chemical thrombolysis and mechanical thrombectomy.[19] In chemical thrombolysis, a microcatheter is advanced through the thrombus via a transvenous approach and a thrombolytic drug, most commonly urokinase or recombinant tissue plasminogen activator (tPA), is infused locally.[19] In mechanical thrombectomy, a stent retriever is used to retrieve the thrombus.[19] Although the transvenous approach to CVST is distinct from the transarterial approach used in acute ischemic stroke, there is crossover with the devices employed.[19] In addition, the success of endovascular treatment for acute ischemic stroke with large vessel occlusion has encouraged the use of this approach in CVST.[13,19]

The literature suggests a recanalization rate of 70% to 90%.[13] Systematic reviews of case series estimate a 10% to 17% rate of new ICH formation after an endovascular procedure.[22–24] The Thrombolysis Or Anticoagulation for Cerebral venous Thrombosis (TO-ACT) trial, comparing standard treatment and endovascular treatment for CVST, was terminated early because of the lack of significant improvement noted at 12 months follow-up.[25] The final results of this trial have not yet been published. However, based on the current evidence, endovascular treatment should not be included in the standard treatment algorithm, but only as a salvage procedure.[13]

INTRACRANIAL PRESSURE MANAGEMENT
Medical

In the event of symptoms secondary to increased ICP, such as with isolated high ICP (nonhemorrhagic) causing headache and threatening vision, the carbonic anhydrase inhibitor acetazolamide may be used in order to decrease CSF production, although the evidence for this treatment is limited.[2,16] Consultation with an ophthalmologist or neuro-ophthalmologist for monitoring of papilledema and visual fields is advisable. If the patient experiences progressive visual loss, then optic nerve decompression, repeated lumbar punctures, or CSF shunting should be considered.[2,13,16]

Surgical

The indications for surgical intervention in CVST are limited to large hemorrhagic infarcts causing significant mass effect and or hydrocephalus.[3,13,14] Decompressive surgery may be performed in patients with clinical or radiographic evidence of impending herniation.[13,16] However, the supporting evidence for the role of surgical decompressive hemicraniectomy in CVST is limited.[13,14,16] A case series published in 2012 included 10 patients who underwent decompressive hemicraniectomy for CVST.[26] In this group, 5 patients achieved a modified Rankin scale (mRS) of 0 to 1 (no disability) at 12 months, and 2 patients succumbed to cerebral edema secondary to expanding venous infarcts.[26] In a second review that included 13 patients published in 2009, 11 patients achieved an mRS of less than 3, which reflects a favorable outcome.[27] Although the level of evidence is limited, previous studies have demonstrated poor patient outcomes in the absence of intervention, and therefore decompressive surgery is recommended for patients with impending herniation.[13,16]

Acute ICP problems with papilledema and visual loss may occasionally require temporizing with an external lumbar drain.[16] Long-term problems with raised ICP can persist, resulting in chronic intracranial hypertension (pseudotumor cerebri), sometimes requiring treatment with a ventriculoperitoneal or lumboperitoneal shunt.[28]

Hydrocephalus occurs in approximately 15% of CVST patients.[13] Most of these patients have thrombosis of the deep venous system and resulting edema of the thalami and basal ganglia that ultimately results in obstructive hydrocephalus.[13] In the advent of increased ICP that is refractory to medical management, neurosurgical consultation should be considered for CSF diversion, in the form of external ventriculostomy or ventriculoperitoneal shunt.[14]

OUTCOME/PROGNOSIS

In contrast to historical beliefs, the long-term prognosis of CVST has improved; still the underlying pathophysiology remains significant, and CVST remains a potentially fatal disease. Approximately one-half of these deaths are caused by the initial precipitating factor, most commonly malignancy, as opposed to the thrombosis itself. In the middle twentieth century, CVST mortality was reported to be between 30% and 50%.[29] Today, mortality in the acute period is approximately 4%.[13] A recent trial of 3488 patients determined a mortality rate of 4.4%.[29] Indicators of poor prognosis include coma on presentation, the extremes of age, deep venous system thrombosis, ICH, CNS infection, and malignancy.[2,13]

Increased awareness of CVST in the medical community and advancements in imaging technology have created a paradigm shift in the prognosis of the disease. However, approximately 80% of individuals do not have lasting significant physical disability from CVST. Approximately 50% report recurrent headaches and neuropsychological effects in follow-up.[13]

SUMMARY

CVST, once considered a rare and fatal disease, now has a more favorable prognosis. These developments are predominantly because of earlier diagnosis and treatment, which have been facilitated by both increased awareness in the medical community and advancements in imaging technology. On that note, it is important to recognize the numerous transient and permanent risk factors associated with CVST, particularly in women of childbearing age. Although anticoagulation is the main treatment, neurosurgical intervention may be needed, including decompressive craniectomy, temporary or permanent shunt insertion, and endovascular procedures such as transvenous injection of thrombolytics or mechanical thrombectomy.

REFERENCES

1. Bousser M-G, Ferro JM. Cerebral venous thrombosis: an update. Lancet Neurol 2007;6(2): 162–70.
2. Demchuk A, Venegas-Torres J. Cranial venous sinus thrombosis diagnosis and management. In: Hamilton M, Golfinos J, Pineo G, et al, editors. Handbook of bleeding and coagulation for neurosurgery. New York: Thieme; 2015. p. 184–96.
3. Stam J. Cerebral venous and sinus thrombosis: incidence and causes. Adv Neurol 2003;92:225–32.
4. Devasagayam S, Wyatt B, Leyden J, et al. Cerebral venous sinus thrombosis incidence is higher than previously thought: a retrospective population-based study. Stroke 2016;47(9):2180–2.
5. Coutinho JM, Zuurbier SM, Aramideh M, et al. The incidence of cerebral venous thrombosis: a cross-sectional study. Stroke 2012;43(12):3375–7.
6. Ferro JM, Canhão P, Stam J, et al. Prognosis of cerebral vein and dural sinus thrombosis: results of the International Study on Cerebral Vein and Dural Sinus Thrombosis (ISCVT). Stroke 2004; 35(3):664–70.
7. Stam J. Thrombosis of the cerebral veins and sinuses. N Engl J Med 2005;353:791–8.
8. de Bruijn SFTM, Stam J, Koopman MMW, et al. Case-control study of risk of cerebral sinus thrombosis in oral contraceptive users who are carriers of hereditary prothrombotic conditions. BMJ 1998; 316(7131):589–92.
9. Cantu C, Barinagarrementeria F. Cerebral venous thrombosis associated with pregnancy and

puerperium. Review of 67 cases. Stroke 1993; 24(12):1880–4.

10. Lanska DJ, Kryscio RJ. Risk factors for peripartum and postpartum stroke and intracranial venous thrombosis. Stroke 2000;31(6):1274–82.

11. Gessler F, Bruder M, Duetzmann S, et al. Risk factors governing the development of cerebral vein and dural sinus thrombosis after craniotomy in patients with intracranial tumors. J Neurosurg 2017; 1–7. https://doi.org/10.3171/2016.11.JNS161871.

12. De Bruijn SFTM, Stam J, Kappelle LJ. Thunderclap headache as first symptom of cerebral venous sinus thrombosis. Lancet 1996;348(9042):1623–5.

13. Silvis SM, De Sousa DA, Ferro JM, et al. Cerebral venous thrombosis. Nat Rev Neurol 2017;13(9): 555–65.

14. Bushnell C, Saposnik G. Evaluation and management of cerebral venous thrombosis. Continuum (Minneap Minn) 2014;20(2):335–51.

15. Saposnik G, Barinagarrementeria F, Brown RD, et al. Diagnosis and management of cerebral venous thrombosis: a statement for healthcare professionals from the American Heart Association/American Stroke Association. Stroke 2011;42(4):1158–92.

16. Ferro JM, Bousser M-G, Canhão P, et al. European Stroke Organization guideline for the diagnosis and treatment of cerebral venous thrombosis - endorsed by the European Academy of Neurology. Eur J Neurol 2017;2(3):195–221.

17. Linn J, Ertl-Wagner B, Seelos KC, et al. Diagnostic value of multidetector-row CT angiography in the evaluation of thrombosis of the cerebral venous sinuses. AJNR Am J Neuroradiol 2007;28(5):946–52.

18. Canhão P, Cortesão A, Cabral M, et al. Are steroids useful to treat cerebral venous thrombosis? Stroke 2008;39(1):105–10.

19. Coutinho J, de Bruijn SF, Deveber G, et al. Anticoagulation for cerebral venous sinus thrombosis. Cochrane Database Syst Rev 2011;(8):CD002005.

20. Erkens PMG, Prins MH. Fixed dose subcutaneous low molecular weight heparins versus adjusted dose unfractionated heparin for venous thromboembolism. Cochrane Database Syst Rev 2010;(9): CD001100.

21. Anticoli S, Pezzella FR, Scifoni G, et al. Treatment of cerebral venous thrombosis with rivaroxaban. J Biomed Sci 2016;5(3). https://doi.org/10.4172/2254-609x.100031.

22. Siddiqui FM, Dandapat S, Banerjee C, et al. Mechanical thrombectomy in cerebral venous thrombosis: systematic review of 185 cases. Stroke 2015;46(5):1263–8.

23. Canhão P, Falcão F, Ferro JM. Thrombolytics for cerebral sinus thrombosis: a systematic review. Cerebrovasc Dis 2003;15(3):159–66.

24. Haghighi AB, Mahmoodi M, Edgell RC, et al. Mechanical thrombectomy for cerebral venous sinus thrombosis. Clin Appl Thromb Hemost 2014;20(5): 507–15.

25. Coutinho JM, Ferro JM, Zuurbier SM, et al. Thrombolysis or anticoagulation for cerebral venous thrombosis: rationale and design of the TO-ACT trial. Int J Stroke 2013;8(2):135–40.

26. Zuurbier SM, Coutinho JM, Majoie CBLM, et al. Decompressive hemicraniectomy in severe cerebral venous thrombosis: a prospective case series. J Neurol 2012;259(6):1099–105.

27. Coutinho JM, Majoie CBLM, Coert BA, et al. Decompressive hemicraniectomy in cerebral sinus thrombosis: consecutive case series and review of the literature. Stroke 2009;40(6):2233–5.

28. Biousse V, Bruce BB, Newman NJ. Update on the pathophysiology and management of idiopathic intracranial hypertension. J Neurol Neurosurg Psychiatry 2012;83(5):488–94.

29. Haghighi AB, Edgell RC, Cruz-Flores S, et al. Mortality of cerebral venous-sinus thrombosis in a large national sample. Stroke 2012;43(1):262–4.

Management of Acute Ischemic Thrombosis

Kunal Vakharia, MD[a], Gursant S. Atwal, MD[a], Elad I. Levy, MD, MBA[a,b,*]

KEYWORDS

- Acute ischemic thrombosis • Occlusive cerebrovascular disease • Stroke
- Intracranial atherosclerotic disease • Perfusion imaging

KEY POINTS

- Noninvasive perfusion imaging has become important for the management of stroke in evaluating time-to-peak, cerebral blood volume, and cerebral blood flow in acute ischemic stroke and penumbra regions.
- Endovascular techniques for acute ischemic thrombosis include aspiration through a large-bore catheter (known as the A Direct Aspiration first Pass Technique [ADAPT]), the use of a stent retriever, and a combination of the 2 techniques (known as Solumbra or Trenumbra).
- Management of acute ischemic thrombosis in neurosurgical patients requires early detection and aggressive intervention. The use of perfusion imaging studies to discern viable tissue is important in understanding the risk–benefit analysis.

INTRODUCTION

The brain is the organ in the body that is most vulnerable to hypoperfusion. Ischemic changes happen quickly because of the demand of the brain for oxygen and glucose. Exclusive aerobic metabolism and high metabolic rates are needed to maintain ionic gradients and constant synaptic activity. This organ comprises only 2% of the human body weight but uses 18% of the cardiac output.[1] Because of this, even small fluctuations generate significant changes in electrochemical gradients and neuronal cell functioning.

Several mechanisms that protect cerebral blood flow (CBF) include multiplicity of supply via collateral blood vessels and the Circle of Willis and physiologic local perfusion matching and autoregulation to areas of increased metabolism. In settings of acute ischemic thrombosis, understanding the dynamic nature of CBF and its relationship to cerebral blood volume (CBV) is crucial in identifying viable brain tissue (salvageable penumbra) that is at risk.[2] In cases of acute ischemic thrombosis, the interventionist must consider physiologic responses of blood vessels and compensatory mechanisms such as autoregulation while trying to improve CBF and CBV.

PATHOPHYSIOLOGY

The 2 most significant pathophysiological causes of acute ischemia are atherosclerotic disease

Disclosure Statement: Dr E.I. Levy has shareholder/ownership interests in Intratech Medical Ltd. and NeXtGen Biologics. He serves as a national primary investigator for the Medtronic US SWIFT PRIME trials and receives honoraria for training and lecturing from that company. He receives compensation from Abbott Vascular for carotid training sessions for physicians. He serves as a consultant to Pulsar Vascular and on the Acute Ischemic Stroke Clinical Advisory Board for Stryker and the Advisory Board for NeXtGen Biologics, MEDX, and Cognition Medical. Dr K. Vakharia and Dr G.S. Atwal have nothing to report.
a Department of Neurosurgery, University at Buffalo, 100 High Street, B4, Buffalo, NY 14203, USA; b Clinical and Translational Research Center, CSRVC, 875 Ellicott Street, Buffalo, NY 14214, USA
* Corresponding author. Department of Neurosurgery, University at Buffalo, 100 High Street, B4, Buffalo, NY 14203.
E-mail address: elevy@ubns.com

Neurosurg Clin N Am 29 (2018) 595–604
https://doi.org/10.1016/j.nec.2018.06.012
1042-3680/18/© 2018 Elsevier Inc. All rights reserved.

and thromboembolism. Low-density lipoproteins (LDLs) and triglycerides play a large role in atherosclerotic disease. The plaque initially forms as a fatty streak secondary to elevated LDL cholesterol deposition that initiates the immune response of macrophages, leading to a proinflammatory state. LDL oxidation leads to incorporation of cholesterol deposits into the subendothelial layer of the blood vessels. Injury to the intimal layer from accumulation of these deposits can cause platelet aggregation and thrombus formation that may lead to stenosis of the vessel.[3] Rupture of plaques can lead to acute ischemic events as well as occlusion at the site of the stenosis.

Another common cause of acute ischemia involves thromboemboli leading to acute occlusions. Atherosclerotic disease of proximal vessels and atrial fibrillation are typical causes of acute ischemia. Both of these causes can potentially lead to thromboemboli, which when distributed more distally, can impede blood flow in the cranial circulation. In addition, other sources of thromboemboli include fusiform aneurysms, arterial wall dissections, trauma-causing blunt vessel injury, traumatic injury to vessels, hypercoagulable states, and postoperative hypercoagulability, all of which contribute to higher risks of acute arterial intracranial thrombosis.[4] Appropriate postoperative anticoagulation for known hypercoagulable states is recommended, typically focusing on antithrombin and antifactor Xa therapies, discussed in other articles in this edition.[5]

In addition to these causes of acute ischemia, surgical procedures that involve manipulation of arteries and endovascular procedures can increase the risk of thromboembolic complications. Surgical bypass procedures, endarterectomies, and other procedures involving manipulation of the intracranial vasculature predispose vessels to arterial thrombosis. Vessel injury, flow stasis, turbulent blood flow, and immobility of the patient can also predispose vessels to thrombosis. Surgeons performing open vascular procedures need to consider the contact of suture lines or surgical material including patch grafts and other grafts with the circulation. Endovascular procedures have an inherent risk of arterial thrombosis of nearly 1% per procedure and up to 5% to 7% for interventions.[6] Antiplatelet therapy can help prevent intraprocedural thrombosis, because the mechanism for thrombosis is believed to be secondary to platelet aggregation. Anticoagulation therapy, including systemic heparinization during procedures, is standard for most endovascular interventions and helps to reduce the risk of thrombosis by acting on the intrinsic coagulation cascade, which may be activated when the plastic or metal components of the endovascular catheters and devices are in contact with blood for extended periods of time.

DIAGNOSIS

Patients with acute arterial thrombosis tend to present with significant symptomatic findings on clinical examination. Symptoms referable to motor and sensory areas of the cortex indicate risk for cerebral ischemia or cerebral hypoperfusion.[7] Even in neurosurgical patients, clinical findings can be localized, and prognosis can be partially understood by determining the National Institutes of Health Stroke Scale (NIHSS) for symptoms that last more than 15 minutes. A baseline neurologic examination and NIHSS score are paramount for patients who undergo neurosurgical procedures, because understanding postoperative changes in clinical findings and the score may play a role in determining whether surgical intervention is warranted.[8]

Initial imaging modalities include noncontrast computed tomography (CT) of the head to exclude intracranial hemorrhage or postoperative causes for the changes in the neurologic examination. Early changes may be noted near the gray–white matter junction, basal ganglia, and insular cortex in nearly 50% of cases.[9,10] The Alberta Stroke Programme Early CT Score (ASPECTS) was established to guide revascularization efforts in acute stroke patients.[9] The ASPECTS investigators found that patients with scores less than 7 were noted to have a higher risk of symptomatic hemorrhage with thrombolytic therapy and lower modified Rankin Scale (mRS) scores at 3 months. Further studies demonstrated the potential importance of CT angiography to demonstrate arterial anatomy and suggest potential targets for revascularization.[2] Thrombolytic therapy for treatment of acute ischemic thrombosis is not a common option in postsurgical patients because of the risk of hemorrhage.

The capabilities of CT angiography were further extended with CT perfusion imaging technology. At the authors' institute, CT perfusion imaging is used to guide endovascular and open vascular revascularization decisions.[11] Determining whether increased time to peak correlates with areas of decreased CBF and CBV can delineate areas of brain that are salvageable versus areas that demonstrate core infarct.[12] The risks of endovascular or surgical revascularization in the presence of a core infarct are concerning because of a higher risk of reperfusion injury and hemorrhage.[13,14] Patients with small areas of core infarct but with a large ischemic penumbra can benefit from prompt surgical intervention.

MRI has also been a useful adjunct in the diagnosis of acute arterial thrombosis. MR images can show areas of completed ischemia and help determine whether intervention is warranted. MR perfusion imaging is used at some institutions to determine if brain tissue is still viable. A subanalysis of patients enrolled in the Solitaire With the Intention For Thrombectomy as PRIMary Endovascular Treatment (SWIFT PRIME) trial failed to chow any additional benefit of using CT perfusion imaging compared with MRI prior to endovascular revascularization therapy.[15]

PROGNOSIS

Prognosis for acute ischemic strokes is an evolving process. Although many imaging modalities have been applied to assess and predict long-term outcomes, this is a process in constant flux. With recent results in the DWI or CTP Assessment with Clinical Mismatch in the Triage of Wake-Up and Late Presenting Strokes Undergoing Neurointervention with Trevo (DAWN) trial, patients with acute stroke who had last been known to be well 6 to 24 hours earlier who had a mismatch between clinical deficit and infarct volume had improved disability outcomes at 90 days if they underwent thrombectomy plus standard care compared with those who underwent standard care alone.[16] The use of perfusion mismatch to determine the utility of endovascular thrombectomy was validated by the Endovascular Therapy Following Imaging Evaluation for Ischemic Core 3 (DEFUSE 3) trial.[17] This trial ran concurrently with DAWN, evaluated patients who presented with ischemic stroke with MRI or CTP 6 to 16 hours after last being known to be well and also demonstrated an improved mRS at 90 days in patients treated with endovascular thrombectomy who presented with a mismatch compared with standard medical care.[17]

Muir and colleagues[2] evaluated 408 patients, including 373 patients with confirmed acute stroke; they completed follow-up, and compared prognosis and prediction based on stroke scoring scales including the NIHSS, the Canadian Neurologic Scale, and the Middle Cerebral Artery Neurologic Score. Each of the 3 scores predicted 3-month outcomes with an accuracy of 0.79 or greater. NIHSS was the most sensitive predictor of poor outcome and overall accuracy. A cutpoint of an NIHSS score of 13 best predicted 3-month outcomes for patients.

With ASPECTS, eloquent regions of the brain that have demonstrated hypodense changes portend a worse prognosis. Although noncontrast CT and MRI modalities cannot be used to determine when to intervene, they can help in long-term prognosis concerning areas of infarct. Puetz and colleagues[18] noted the difficulty in discerning prognosis of posterior circulation arterial thrombosis on CT angiography source images. They found that the extent of hypoattenuation on these images served as a good predictor of functional outcome in patients with basilar artery occlusions and posterior circulation strokes. With increasing use of CT perfusion imaging, more advanced methods of determining core, viable areas, and areas that may benefit from other surgical revascularization techniques versus flow augmentation will become increasingly relevant.[19]

CLINICAL MANAGEMENT

Patients with acute arterial thrombosis require substantial and urgent care. The 2015 American Heart Association and American Stroke Association Focused Update of 2013 Guidelines for the management of acute ischemic stroke recommended intravenous recombinant tissue plasminogen activator (IV-tPA) for patients within a 4.5-hour window from symptom onset.[20] This therapy resulted in improved functional outcome at 3 and 6 months. The guidelines note that there is a 6.4% rate of hemorrhagic complication in patients who have undergone recent surgical procedures; for these patients, IV-tPA administration remains a contraindication.[21] This poses a challenging risk-benefit assessment for clinicians regarding postoperative patients, especially neurosurgical patients. Patients most at risk of acute arterial thrombosis in the neurosurgical population include those who recently underwent an extracranial or an intracranial vascular procedure, those of limited mobility, or those who become hypercoagulable, such as oncology patients.

In postoperative patients, a change in neurologic examination findings should prompt noncontrast CT imaging. This imaging will help the clinician recognize postoperative complications, hematoma formation, or other nonarterial complications. CT and MR perfusion imaging are used to discern ischemic penumbra, and CT angiography helps determine targets for possible intervention.[22] An immediate return to the endovascular suite or operating room may be warranted for patients who exhibit acute neurologic changes postprocedurally.

Patients undergoing procedures on extracranial vessels include those undergoing endovascular or open surgical intervention on carotid or vertebral arteries. Although it has become standard practice to use embolic protection devices, patients undergoing endovascular intervention may have acute ischemic symptoms secondary to plaque disruption and distal arterial-to-arterial emboli. Dual antiplatelet therapy tends to help stabilize plaque morphology. For endovascular procedures, IV-tPA may be warranted in the acute setting. For patients who have undergone open surgical intervention, such as a carotid endarterectomy, there should be a low threshold to re-explore the surgical site if patients present with neurologic deficits immediately postprocedurally. This is largely because of the higher risk of immediate thromboembolism from the suture site or immediately distal to the suture site into the petrous portion of the carotid artery because of the clamp time.[23,24] Intra-arterial thrombosis along the suture line or immediately distal to the surgical site poses a known risk to intervention. **Fig. 1** shows the images of a patient who underwent carotid endarterectomy and, on the same day, presented with an NIHSS score of 12 and ischemic symptoms after the initial procedure. The patient was found to have an arterial thrombus at the endarterectomy site and was taken to the operating room for

surgical site exploration. Suction aspiration was used to evacuate a large clot from the cervicopetrous carotid artery and re-establish flow. Suction aspiration of the arteriotomy and the use of a Fogarty balloon-tip catheter (Edwards Lifesciences, Irvine California) inserted intra-arterially to the skull base can be used as techniques to access distal occlusions and improve recanalization rates during such interventions.

Patients undergoing intracranial vascular procedures have a similar complication profile. Open surgical manipulation of blood vessels and perivessel bipolar coagulation can predispose vessels to arterial thrombus formation and vasospasm. Patients with acute hemorrhage pose a secondary risk of progressive hemorrhage and further complications when antiplatelet therapy or anticoagulation is administered. Direct surgical and endovascular interventions tend to be the best options. **Fig. 2** shows the images of a patient who presented with an acute posterior communicating artery aneurysm rupture who underwent open surgical evacuation of the clot (**Fig. 2**A) and clip

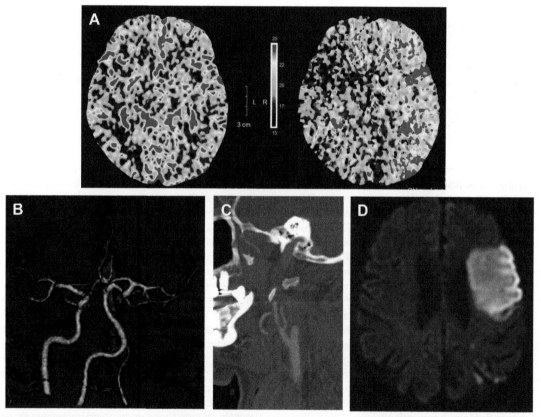

Fig. 1. (*A*) CT perfusion images show an abnormality in the left middle cerebral artery (MCA) distribution with preserved cerebral blood volume indicating salvageable penumbra. (*B*) CT angiography reconstruction shows left internal carotid artery (ICA) occlusion with cross filling via the anterior communicating artery. (*C*) Sagittal CT angiography reconstruction shows a left cervical ICA occlusion. (*D*) Postoperative magnetic resonance (MR) image shows an area of completed infarct.

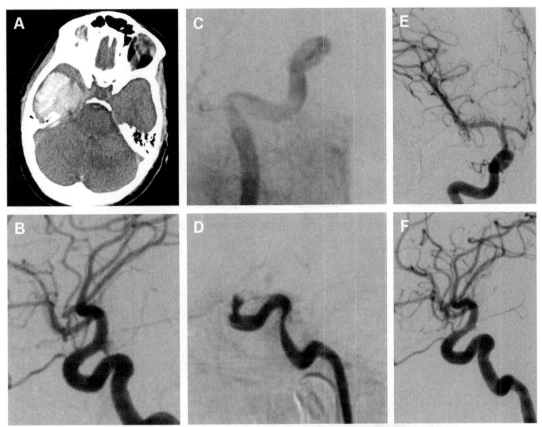

Fig. 2. (*A*) Noncontrast CT scan of the head displays a right temporal lobe hematoma. (*B*) Digital subtraction angiogram (DSA), right ICA injection, lateral view shows a posterior communicating artery aneurysm. Digital subtraction angiogram, right ICA injection, anteroposterior (AP) (*C*) and lateral (*D*) views show postcraniotomy ICA occlusion. Digital subtraction angiogram, right ICA injection, AP (*E*) and lateral (*F*) views, shows complete recanalization post-thrombectomy.

ligation of the aneurysm (see **Fig. 2**B). Postprocedurally, the patient was found to have a worsening neurologic examination, and perfusion imaging showed increased time to peak and preserved CBV in the right internal carotid artery (ICA) distribution, indicating salvageable penumbra. Angiography demonstrated right ICA occlusion (**Fig. 2**C, D). The patient was taken for emergent thrombectomy, and complete recanalization was achieved using an aspiration catheter (ADAPT) (**Fig. 2**E, F). Although vessels around the surgical site are believed to be more tenuous after a recent surgical intervention, large vessels such as the supraclinoid ICA have proven to be robust and allow for endovascular intervention with stent retrievers or aspiration catheters.[23,25]

In addition, patients undergoing endovascular intervention can be at risk of arterial thrombosis. **Fig. 3** communicates a case in which a patient presented with a subacute right temporal lobe hemorrhage and was found to have an arteriovenous malformation (AVM). During preoperative Onyx

(Medtronic, Minneapolis, Minnesota) embolization of one of the arterial pedicles, the microcatheter was stuck and left in situ. Following the stroke protocol at the authors' institute, the patient was placed on a heparin drip overnight that was discontinued 4 hours prior to surgery. The catheter was removed during the resection of the AVM. Despite the removal of the microcatheter, the patient had an acute arterial thrombus recognized by an acute change in the neurologic examination. Perfusion imaging showed salvageable penumbra (see **Fig. 3**E), and he was taken for emergent thrombectomy for right MCA occlusion (see **Fig. 3**F), which resulted in complete recanalization (see **Fig. 3**G, H). Early recognition and treatment of occlusive intracranial disease are critical and led to good outcomes in these patients.

Although procedures requiring direct manipulation of blood vessels predispose patients to acute arterial thrombosis and vasospasm, it is important to understand that patients who have undergone surgical intervention for spinal or oncological

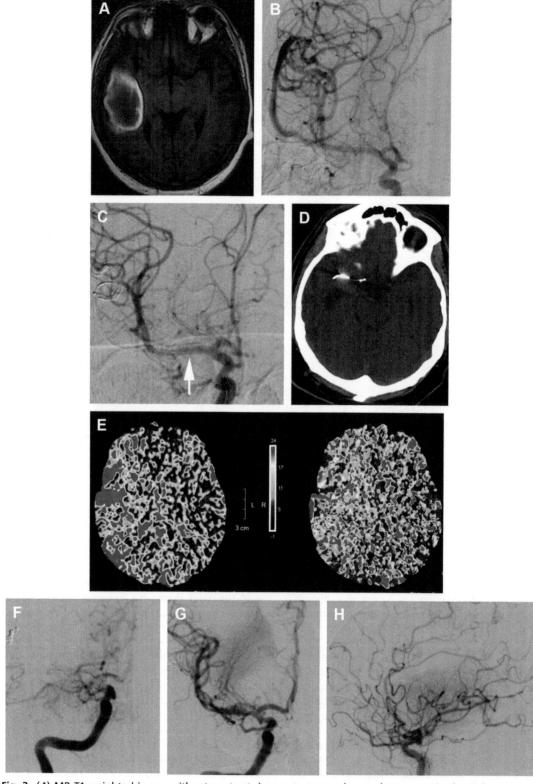

Fig. 3. (*A*) MR T1-weighted image without contrast demonstrates a subacute hematoma in the right temporal lobe. (*B*) DSA, right ICA injection, AP view shows a right temporal arteriovenous malformation fed by MCA branches. (*C*) DSA, right ICA injection, AP view shows Onyx (Medtronic, Minneapolis Minnesota) embolization

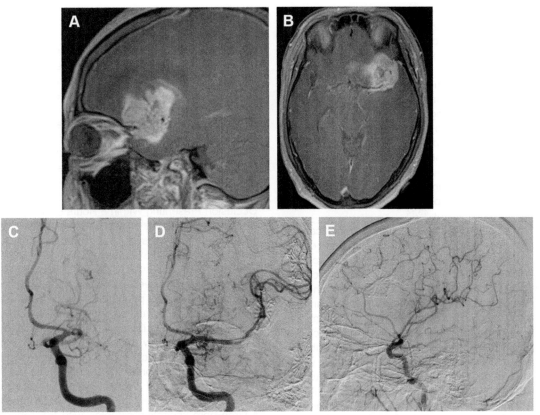

Fig. 4. (*A*) Sagittal view of MR T1-weighted image with contrast demonstrates left frontotemporal tumor involving the left middle cerebral artery (MCA). (*B*) Axial view of MR T1-weighted image with contrast demonstrates left frontotemporal tumor involving the left MCA. (*C*) DSA, left ICA injection, AP view showing left M1 occlusion. Digital subtraction angiogram, left ICA injection, AP (*D*) and lateral (*E*) views showing thrombolysis in cerebral infarction grade 2b recanalization post-thrombectomy.

procedures are also at a heightened risk. Perry and colleagues and multiple meta-analyses have demonstrated the increased risk of venous and arterial thromboembolic complications in glioma patients.[26,27] Fraum and colleagues[26] demonstrated that patients on antiangiogenic medications have a nearly 50% risk of ischemic stroke in a small study population. Given these findings, understanding the need for anticoagulation and prophylaxis in these patients is critical. **Fig. 4** is an example of a patient who underwent a left craniotomy for resection of a frontotemporal glioblastoma and presented with acute left MCA syndrome. Six days postoperatively, the patient was noted to have acute onset of global aphasia,

right-sided hemiplegia, and hemineglect. MR perfusion imaging showed increased time-to-peak with a small area of loss of CBV, and a large area of penumbra. Vascular imaging showed left MCA occlusion. Cases such as this are difficult and pose challenges to possible interventional modalities. Although there are no large studies for validation, understanding the fragility of vessels within and around postsurgical sites is important. Thrombolytic therapies are not an option for these patients, and stent retrievers can pose significant risks to the intima of medium-sized vessels that have been recently manipulated.[28,29] In such cases, the use of aspiration alone (ADAPT) can be useful to minimize trauma to the intima. In this

---

with retained microcatheter (*arrow*). (*D*) Postembolization noncontrast CT scan of the head demonstrating retained microcatheter in the sylvian fissure (*arrow*). (*E*) CT perfusion images show perfusion abnormality in the right MCA distribution with preserved cerebral blood volume indicating salvageable penumbra. (*F*) DSA, right ICA injection, AP view demonstrates right MCA occlusion. DSA, right ICA injection, AP (*G*) and Lateral (*H*) views demonstrating complete recanalization post thrombectomy.

patient, aspiration thrombectomy was performed, with partial recanalization achieved.

After thrombectomy, neurosurgical patients need to be monitored closely in the intensive care unit. Risks of recurrent stroke, post-thrombectomy hemorrhage, and strict management of blood pressure parameters become vitally important. Following thrombectomy, a noncontrast CT scan is obtained to look for contrast extravasation and possible risks of hemorrhage, which help dictate blood pressure management.[14] Typically, permissive hypertension to systolic blood pressures under 180 mm Hg allows for improved cerebral perfusion while limiting hemorrhagic complications.[13,14]

In addition to these ischemic complications, there are disease subtypes that also pose certain risks for the development of acute ischemic thrombosis. Moyamoya disease and its ischemic complications are well recognized. Although direct external carotid-to-ICA bypass grafts can help augment anterior circulation flow in these patients, these grafts tend to have complications of their own. Natarajan and colleagues[30] described a case of a patient with Moyamoya disease whose direct bypass had occluded, which led to new ischemic symptoms and a perfusion deficit. This patient was treated with a second bypass from the patent vessel graft to the intracranial circulation and had improved perfusion on 5-month follow-up. Of note, bypass vessels tend to be tenuous and prone to spasm, making antispasmodic therapy an important preparation for manipulation of these vessels.

TECHNIQUES

Endovascular techniques for revascularization have significantly improved over the years. Retrievable stent technology demonstrated significant superiority in recanalization for acute arterial thrombosis.[31–33] A stent retriever is a self-expanding stent used to retrieve the thromboembolus and restore blood flow.[31] Current techniques for mechanical thrombectomy involve what has been termed the tower of power, which is a triaxial system comprised of a guide catheter, an intermediate catheter, a microcatheter with a microwire, and a stent retriever that can be deployed distally and retrieved to allow for effective recanalization. The intermediate or aspiration catheter can be used as an adjunct to the stent retriever. A combination of these techniques (Solumbra or Trenumbra technique) is most often used and limits the pull on the intima of the vessel while attempting to suction debris from the thrombectomy with an aspiration catheter.[28]

EVIDENCE

The 5 stent retriever trials include a multicenter randomized clinical trial of endovascular treatment for acute ischemic stroke in the Netherlands (MR CLEAN),[31] The Endovascular Treatment for Small Core and Anterior Circulation Proximal Occlusion with Emphasis on Minimizing CT to Recanalization Times (ESCAPE),[32] Extending the Time for Thrombolysis in Emergency Neurologic Deficits—Intra-Arterial (EXTEND-IA),[6] Randomized Trial of Revascularization With Solitaire FR Device versus Best Medical Therapy in the Treatment of Acute Stroke Due to Anterior Circulation Large Vessel Occlusion Presenting Within 8 Hours of Symptom Onset (REVASCAT),[34] and SWIFT PRIME.[35] Together, these trials showed improved clinical outcomes, with an 88% recanalization rate noted in large-vessel occlusions. The time window for thrombectomy has been extended using perfusion imaging to evaluate penumbra versus ischemic core to guide intervention in both DAWN and DEFUSE 3.[16,17] Results of the DAWN trial have extended this window to up to 24 hours.[16] The comparison of direct aspiration versus stent retriever as a first approach (COMPASS) trial evaluated stent retrieval versus primary aspiration alone.[36] Primary aspiration is carried out through a large-bore aspiration catheter, with the aspiration catheter advanced to the proximal face of the clot, and suction applied. The absence of flow in the aspiration pump indicates occlusion and optimal apposition against the clot interface. Aspiration is applied for 3 minutes prior to withdrawing the system. This method tends to be less traumatic to distal vessels, largely by not injuring the intima. The drawback to this technique is that it can be harder to advance the aspiration catheter into more distal vessels including the M2 and M3 MCA segments, where stent retrievers and 3-dimensional stent retrievers can sometimes be deployed. In a large multicenter prospective study, Turk and colleagues[29] found that the ADAPT had a 78% recanalization rate in large vessel occlusions, with thrombolysis in cerebral infarction (TICI) 2B and TICI 3 outcomes.

SUMMARY

Acute arterial thrombosis can lead to devastating morbidity. Early recognition and intervention are key to achieving good clinical outcomes. Advances in endovascular techniques for mechanical thrombectomy have improved outcomes in acute ischemic stroke as evidenced by multiple randomized trials. Additionally, CT perfusion imaging is critical in evaluating tissue at risk and is our preferred modality for evaluating patients with acute neurologic deterioration who have a negative noncontrast CT scan. Open neurosurgical patients are unlikely to be candidates for thrombolytic therapies. However, in endovascular neurosurgical patients, thrombolytic therapy may improve outcomes in small-vessel ischemia.

REFERENCES

1. Attwell D, Buchan AM, Charpak S, et al. Glial and neuronal control of brain blood flow. Nature 2010; 468:232–43.
2. Muir KW, Weir CJ, Murray GD, et al. Comparison of neurological scales and scoring systems for acute stroke prognosis. Stroke 1996;27:1817–20.
3. Puddu P, Puddu GM, Bastagli L, et al. Coronary and cerebrovascular atherosclerosis: two aspects of the same disease or two different pathologies? Arch Gerontol Geriatr 1995;20:15–22.
4. Rincon F, Sacco RL, Kranwinkel G, et al. Incidence and risk factors of intracranial atherosclerotic stroke: the Northern Manhattan Stroke Study. Cerebrovasc Dis 2009;28:65–71.
5. Chimowitz MI, Lynn MJ, Howlett-Smith H, et al. Comparison of warfarin and aspirin for symptomatic intracranial arterial stenosis. N Engl J Med 2005; 352:1305–16.
6. Campbell BC, Mitchell PJ, Kleinig TJ, et al. Endovascular therapy for ischemic stroke with perfusion-imaging selection. N Engl J Med 2015; 372:1009–18.
7. Komotar RJ, Wilson DA, Mocco J, et al. Natural history of intracranial atherosclerosis: a critical review. Neurosurgery 2006;58:595–601 [discussion: 595–601].
8. Brott T, Adams HP Jr, Olinger CP, et al. Measurements of acute cerebral infarction: a clinical examination scale. Stroke 1989;20:864–70.
9. Barber PA, Demchuk AM, Zhang J, et al. Validity and reliability of a quantitative computed tomography score in predicting outcome of hyperacute stroke before thrombolytic therapy. ASPECTS Study Group. Alberta Stroke Programme Early CT Score. Lancet 2000;355:1670–4.
10. von Kummer R, Bourquain H, Bastianello S, et al. Early prediction of irreversible brain damage after ischemic stroke at CT. Radiology 2001;219:95–100.
11. Mokin M, Morr S, Fanous AA, et al. Correlation between cerebral blood volume values and outcomes in endovascular therapy for acute ischemic stroke. J Neurointerv Surg 2015;7:705–8.
12. Hirai T, Korogi Y, Ono K, et al. Prospective evaluation of suspected stenoocclusive disease of the intracranial artery: combined MR angiography and CT angiography compared with digital subtraction angiography. AJNR Am J Neuroradiol 2002;23:93–101.
13. Heck DV, Brown MD. Carotid stenting and intracranial thrombectomy for treatment of acute stroke due to tandem occlusions with aggressive antiplatelet therapy may be associated with a high incidence of intracranial hemorrhage. J Neurointerv Surg 2015; 7:170–5.
14. Jain AR, Jain M, Kanthala AR, et al. Association of CT perfusion parameters with hemorrhagic transformation in acute ischemic stroke. AJNR Am J Neuroradiol 2013;34:1895–900.
15. Menjot de Champfleur N, Saver JL, Goyal M, et al. Efficacy of stent-retriever thrombectomy in magnetic resonance imaging versus computed tomographic perfusion-selected patients in SWIFT PRIME trial (Solitaire FR With the Intention for Thrombectomy as Primary Endovascular Treatment for Acute Ischemic Stroke). Stroke 2017;48:1560–6.
16. Nogueira RG, Jadhav AP, Haussen DC, et al, for the DAWN Trial Investigators. Thrombectomy 6 to 24 hours after stroke with a mismatch between deficit and infarct. N Engl J Med 2018;378:11–21.
17. Albers GW, Marks MP, Kemp S, et al, for the DEFUSE 3 Trial Investigators. Thrombectomy for stroke at 6 to 16 hours with selection by perfusion imaging. N Engl J Med 2018;378:708–18.
18. Puetz V, Sylaja PN, Coutts SB, et al. Extent of hypoattenuation on CT angiography source images predicts functional outcome in patients with basilar artery occlusion. Stroke 2008;39:2485–90.
19. Wildermuth S, Knauth M, Brandt T, et al. Role of CT angiography in patient selection for thrombolytic therapy in acute hemispheric stroke. Stroke 1998; 29:935–8.
20. Powers WJ, Derdeyn CP, Biller J, et al. 2015 American Heart Association/American Stroke Association focused update of the 2013 guidelines for the early management of patients with acute ischemic stroke regarding endovascular treatment: a guideline for healthcare professionals from the American Heart Association/American Stroke Association. Stroke 2015;46:3020–35.
21. Furlan AJ, Eyding D, Albers GW, et al. Dose Escalation of Desmoteplase for Acute Ischemic Stroke (DEDAS): evidence of safety and efficacy 3 to 9 hours after stroke onset. Stroke 2006;37:1227–31.
22. Verro P, Tanenbaum LN, Borden NM, et al. CT angiography in acute ischemic stroke: preliminary results. Stroke 2002;33:276–8.
23. Ciccone A, Valvassori L. Endovascular treatment for acute ischemic stroke. N Engl J Med 2013;368: 2433–4.
24. Tong E, Hou Q, Fiebach JB, et al. The role of imaging in acute ischemic stroke. Neurosurg Focus 2014; 36:E3.
25. Penumbra Pivotal Stroke Investigators. The Penumbra pivotal stroke trial: safety and effectiveness of a new generation of mechanical devices for clot

removal in intracranial large vessel occlusive disease. Stroke 2009;40:2761–8.

26. Fraum TJ, Kreisl TN, Sul J, et al. Ischemic stroke and intracranial hemorrhage in glioma patients on antiangiogenic therapy. J Neurooncol 2011;105: 281–9.

27. Perry JR. Thromboembolic disease in patients with high-grade glioma. Neuro Oncol 2012;14(Suppl 4): iv73–80.

28. Dumont TM, Mokin M, Sorkin GC, et al. Aspiration thrombectomy in concert with stent thrombectomy. J Neurointerv Surg 2014;6:e26.

29. Turk AS, Frei D, Fiorella D, et al. ADAPT FAST study: a direct aspiration first pass technique for acute stroke thrombectomy. J Neurointerv Surg 2014;6: 260–4.

30. Natarajan SK, Hauck EF, Hopkins LN, et al. Endovascular management of symptomatic spasm of radial artery bypass graft: technical case report. Neurosurgery 2010;67:794–8 [discussion: 798].

31. Berkhemer OA, Fransen PS, Beumer D, et al. A randomized trial of intraarterial treatment for acute ischemic stroke. N Engl J Med 2015;372:11–20.

32. Goyal M, Demchuk AM, Menon BK, et al. Randomized assessment of rapid endovascular treatment of ischemic stroke. N Engl J Med 2015;372:1019–30.

33. Hacke W, Donnan G, Fieschi C, et al. Association of outcome with early stroke treatment: pooled analysis of ATLANTIS, ECASS, and NINDS rt-PA stroke trials. Lancet 2004;363:768–74.

34. Jovin TG, Chamorro A, Cobo E, et al. Thrombectomy within 8 hours after symptom onset in ischemic stroke. N Engl J Med 2015;372:2296–306.

35. Saver JL, Goyal M, Bonafe A, et al, for the SWIFT PRIME Investigators. Stent-retriever thrombectomy after intravenous t-PA vs. t-PA alone in stroke. N Engl J Med 2015;372:2285–95.

36. Turk AS, Siddiqui AH, Mocco J. A comparison of direct aspiration versus stent retriever as a first approach ('COMPASS'): protocol. J Neurointerv Surg 2018. [Epub ahead of print].

Management of Intracranial Hemorrhage in the Anticoagulated Patient

Robert Loch Macdonald, MD, PhD, FRCSC[a,b,*]

KEYWORDS

- Anticoagulation • Antiplatelet • Intracranial hemorrhage • Intracerebral hemorrhage
- Subdural hemorrhage • Thrombosis

KEY POINTS

- Anticoagulant drugs should be reversed emergently or urgently in all patients with intracranial hemorrhage and certainly in those requiring surgery.
- If surgery is not planned or can be delayed, then in selected patients who are in good neurologic condition and on short-acting or difficult-to-reverse anticoagulants, it may be reasonable to wait for spontaneous recovery from anticoagulation.
- There is a paucity of data to guide practitioners on whether to reverse antiplatelet drugs in patients with intracranial hemorrhage, but generally it is recommended to not administer platelets.
- Laboratory monitoring should guide the adequacy of reversal for all agents.
- The decision of when and whether to resume anticoagulant and antiplatelet drugs following intracranial hemorrhage requires individualized assessment of the risks of hemorrhage if they are resumed, estimated benefit of the drugs, and thromboembolic risk.

INTRODUCTION

The use of antithrombotic agents, either antiplatelet or anticoagulant drugs, is increasing secondary to the increasing human longevity, diagnosis, and treatment of atrial fibrillation and prevalence of risk factors for atherosclerosis and thromboembolism.[1] There are 6 million Americans on anticoagulants or about 2% of the population, who are at increased risk of intracranial hemorrhage (**Table 1**).[2] Single or dual antiplatelet therapy (DAPT) is the standard of care for patients with acute coronary syndromes and for primary and secondary prevention of cardiovascular events.[3,4] Anticoagulation also is standard of care for prevention and treatment of venous thromboembolism (VTE) in patients with atrial fibrillation at high risk of thromboembolism and in many patients with valvular heart disease.[5,6]

Intracranial hemorrhage may be traumatic or spontaneous. Almost all epidural hematomas are secondary to trauma, whereas all other types of intracranial hemorrhage (acute and chronic subdural hematoma [SDH], subarachnoid hemorrhage [SAH], intracerebral hemorrhage [ICH], intraventricular hemorrhage) may be traumatic or

Disclosures: Dr R.L. Macdonald receives grant support from the Physicians' Services Incorporated Foundation, Brain Aneurysm Foundation and Ontario Genomics/Genome Canada.

[a] Division of Neurosurgery, Department of Surgery, St. Michael's Hospital, Labatt Family Centre of Excellence in Brain Injury and Trauma Research, Keenan Research Centre for Biomedical Science, Li Ka Shing Knowledge Institute, St. Michael's Hospital, University of Toronto, 30 Bond Street, Toronto, Ontario M5B 1W8, Canada;
[b] Department of Physiology, St. Michael's Hospital, Labatt Family Centre of Excellence in Brain Injury and Trauma Research, Keenan Research Centre for Biomedical Science, Li Ka Shing Knowledge Institute, St. Michael's Hospital, University of Toronto, 30 Bond Street, Toronto, Ontario M5B 1W8, Canada
* Division of Neurosurgery, St. Michael's Hospital, 30 Bond Street, Toronto, Ontario M5B 1W8, Canada.
E-mail address: macdonaldlo@smh.ca

Neurosurg Clin N Am 29 (2018) 605–613
https://doi.org/10.1016/j.nec.2018.06.013
1042-3680/18/© 2018 Elsevier Inc. All rights reserved.

Table 1
Indications for anticoagulant and antiplatelet drugs

Generic Name	Indications
Acetylsalicylic acid (aspirin)	Temporary relief of minor aches and pains. Actual most common uses are prevention of cardiovascular disease in men 45 to 79 years of age and women 55 to 79 years of age when benefits due to reduction in myocardial infarction outweigh risks of gastrointestinal bleeding. Includes acute myocardial infarction and those with prior myocardial infarction and angina. Prevention of cardiovascular events in patients with prior stroke or transient ischemic attack. Treatment of signs and symptoms of several rheumatologic diseases.
Dipyridamole	As an alternative to exercise for thallium myocardial perfusion imaging. Other indications are variable but may include in addition to aspirin or warfarin for some patients with prosthetic heart valves or other valvular heart disease and perioperatively in addition to aspirin in patients undergoing cardiac bypass.
Ticlopidine	Reduce the risk of thrombotic stroke in patients allergic to or who have failed on aspirin, prevent coronary artery stent thrombosis in combination with aspirin in the first 2 weeks after placement.
Clopidogrel	Reduce the risk of myocardial infarction and stroke in patients with non-ST segment elevation acute coronary syndrome or myocardial infarction, ST segment elevation myocardial infarction, recent myocardial infarction, stroke, or peripheral artery disease.
Prasugrel	Reduction of thrombotic cardiovascular events (including stent thrombosis) in patients with acute coronary syndrome who are to be managed with percutaneous coronary intervention as follows: patients with unstable angina or non-ST segment elevation myocardial infarction and patients with ST segment elevation myocardial infarction when managed with either primary or delayed percutaneous coronary intervention.
Ticagrelor	Reduce the risk of cardiovascular death, myocardial infarction, and stroke in patients with acute coronary syndrome or myocardial infarction.
Warfarin	Prophylaxis and treatment of venous thrombosis and its extension, pulmonary embolism. Prophylaxis and treatment of thromboembolic complications associated with atrial fibrillation and/or cardiac valve replacement. Reduction in the risk of death, recurrent myocardial infarction, and thromboembolic events such as stroke or systemic embolization after myocardial infarction.
Heparin	Acute treatment of venous thromboembolism, prevention of venous thromboembolism, treatment of acute coronary syndromes including percutaneous coronary interventions, ST segment elevation myocardial infarction, unstable angina/ST segment elevation myocardial infarction. Maintain patency of intravenous, peripheral venous and intra-arterial catheters.
Low molecular weight heparins (enoxaparin, dalteparin)	Prophylaxis and treatment of venous thromboembolism, treatment of angina and non-Q wave/non- ST segment elevation myocardial infarction in patients receiving aspirin, acute ST segment elevation myocardial infarction with or without percutaneous coronary intervention.
Dabigatran	To reduce the risk of stroke and systemic embolism in patients with nonvalvular atrial fibrillation. For the treatment of deep venous thrombosis and pulmonary embolism in patients who have been treated with a parenteral anticoagulant for 5 to 10 days. To reduce the risk of recurrence of deep venous thrombosis and pulmonary embolism in patients who have been previously treated. For the prophylaxis of deep venous thrombosis and pulmonary embolism in patients who have undergone hip replacement surgery.
Argatroban	Indicated as an anticoagulant in patients with or at risk for heparin-induced thrombocytopenia undergoing percutaneous coronary intervention.
Rivaroxaban	Reduce the risk of stroke and systemic embolism in patients with nonvalvular atrial fibrillation. For the prophylaxis of deep vein thrombosis, which may lead to pulmonary embolism in patients undergoing knee or hip replacement surgery.

(continued on next page)

Table 1 *(continued)*	
Generic Name	**Indications**
Edoxaban	Treatment of deep vein thrombosis and pulmonary embolism following 5 to 10 days of initial therapy with a parenteral anticoagulant.
Apixaban	Reduce the risk of stroke and systemic embolism in patients with nonvalvular atrial fibrillation. For the prophylaxis of deep vein thrombosis, which may lead to pulmonary embolism, in patients who have undergone hip or knee replacement surgery. For the treatment of deep vein thrombosis and pulmonary embolism and for the reduction in the risk of recurrent deep vein thrombosis and pulmonary embolism following initial therapy.

spontaneous. Factors to consider in a patient with intracranial hemorrhage who is taking antithrombotic drugs include the history and neurologic condition, the etiology and location of the hemorrhage, laboratory evaluation of the platelet and coagulation system, and details and indications for the antithrombotic drugs. Stopping with or without reversal of the drug effects and then when and if to resume the antithrombotic drugs also need to be considered. There are few randomized clinical trials and thus, little Level 1 evidence to guide practice in these patients. Much of the management is empiric and based on expert opinion.

TRAUMATIC INTRACRANIAL HEMORRHAGE

Anticoagulant and antiplatelet drugs are thought to increase the risk of intracranial hemorrhage and morbidity and mortality in patients who have a traumatic brain injury (TBI).[7] The overall quality of evidence to support this contention, while it seems to be logical, is low and sparse. In general, the effects of these drugs correlate with the degree to which they impair hemostasis and thrombosis, with anticoagulants and warfarin (vitamin K antagonist [VKA]) in turn more than non-VKA oral anticoagulants (NOAC), more dangerous than antiplatelet drugs, and clopidogrel more associated with hemorrhage than aspirin. However, a review of literature addressing the risk of traumatic ICH while on antiplatelet drugs did not find strong evidence to support the idea that these patients are at higher risk of hemorrhage than people not taking antiplatelet drugs.[7] Batchelor and Grayson[7] conducted a meta-analysis evaluating the effects of aspirin or clopidogrel on mortality after blunt TBI. The common odds ratio for mortality among 4 studies of aspirin and 4 of clopidogrel was 2.4 (95% confidence interval [CI]: 0.64–9.3). Thus, there was a statistically insignificant increased risk of death in patients with blunt TBI taking preinjury antiplatelet drugs.

On the other hand, anticoagulant drugs were associated with an increased risk of intracranial hemorrhage in patients with mild TBI.[8] Numerous studies found that patients with TBI who are taking anticoagulant drugs have larger initial intracranial hemorrhages, a higher incidence of delayed hematoma expansion, and higher morbidity and mortality.[9] Meta-analysis of studies of anticoagulant drugs and TBI reported the odds ratio for death was 2.0 (95% CI: 1.6–2.5) for patients anticoagulated before TBI compared with those who were not.[10]

Probably the most studied trauma group is comprised of patients with chronic SDH, recognizing that perhaps only half of these patients recall a history of trauma. Multiple retrospective case series and some cohort studies suggest patients taking antiplatelet and anticoagulant drugs are at increased risk of developing a chronic SDH.[11] Patients on antithrombotic drugs with an acute or chronic SDH are thought to be at higher likelihood of presenting with larger hematomas and more severe neurologic deficits.[12,13]

Furthermore, if anticoagulant drugs are resumed after treating the chronic SDH, there may be an increased risk of recurrent chronic SDH.[14] This risk seems to be nonexistent or at least very low for resumption of antiplatelet drugs other than dual antiplatelet drug therapy, which probably does increase the risk.

SPONTANEOUS INTRACRANIAL HEMORRHAGE

The most common locations of spontaneous intracranial hemorrhage are ICH, followed by SDH (which is variable depending on how chronic SDH is classified) and then SAH. This order of frequency roughly corresponds to that of hemorrhages occurring in patients taking VKA or NOAC. Spontaneous SAH is uncommon in general, and as a result, very uncommon in patients taking anticoagulant drugs. In 1 retrospective study of 480 patients with aneurysmal SAH, 4% were taking anticoagulant drugs before the SAH.[15] The neurologic condition on admission was worse in anticoagulated patients, although after adjusting for this, there was no difference in outcome compared with patients not taking anticoagulant drugs. Among 11,549 patients who had an aneurysm repair procedure and SAH in the National Inpatient Sample, 245 patients (2%) were recorded as being on aspirin prior to hemorrhage and 108 patients (0.9%) on anticoagulant drugs.[16] This sample has many limitations and does not include data on neurologic grade (the most important prognostic factor for outcome), but adjusting for various surrogate measures in multivariate analysis suggested that patients on anticoagulants or aspirin had the same in-hospital mortality as patients not taking these drugs.

Most spontaneous intracranial hemorrhages associated with anticoagulation are ICH, which is consistent with the overall frequency of spontaneous ICH.[17] Second is SDH. Also most data on the risk of ICH with anticoagulant drugs are derived from patients with atrial fibrillation, as this is the main indication for long-term anticoagulation. Some of the considerations here are the risk of morbidity and mortality from untreated atrial fibrillation versus the risks and benefits of prophylaxis and treatment with warfarin or NOACs, all of which have much high-level evidence for quantification of these variables. The risks of untreated atrial fibrillation have been studied and several grading systems developed, including the $CHAD_2$ (1 point for heart failure, hypertension, age >75, diabetes, and 2 points for history of stroke or transient ischemic attack [TIA]) and variants such as CHA_2DS_2-VASc.[18,19] There is a high risk for thromboembolism in patients with mechanical heart valves, atrial fibrillation with high $CHAD_2$ (>=4) or CHA_2DS_2-VASc (>= 6), and recent, unprovoked, recurrent, or cancer-associated venous thromboembolism (VTE). The main risk of anticoagulation is hemorrhage, the risk of which can be assessed using $HEMORR_2HAGES$, HAS-BLED (hypertension, abnormal renal/hepatic function, stroke, bleeding history or predisposition, labile international normalized ratio [INR], >65-years old, drugs/alcohol concomitantly [1 point each] >= 3), and ATRIA scores.[18,20,21]

The risk/benefit of factor Xa inhibitors was assessed in a meta-analysis of 13 clinical trials that randomized 67,688 patients.[22] These drugs significantly reduced the risk of stroke and systemic embolic events compared with warfarin in patients with atrial fibrillation while also reducing the risk of intracranial hemorrhage and all-cause mortality. A randomized clinical trial compared warfarin and 2 doses of dabigatran in 18,113 patients with atrial fibrillation.[17] After a mean follow-up of 2 years, 153 patients had intracranial hemorrhage. Forty-six percent of cases were ICH; 45% of cases were subdural, and 8% of cases were SAH. Dabigatran was associated with a lower risk of traumatic ICH compared with warfarin. Mortality was about twice as high in patients with spontaneous compared with traumatic ICH. The yearly risk of ICH with warfarin was 0.76%, more than double the risk with dabigatran. Meta-analysis of clinical trials comparing warfarin with NOACs found all 3 NOACs available in the United States (rivaroxaban, epixaban, dabigatran) were associated with a lower risk of ICH than warfarin.[23]

PATIENT EVALUATION OVERVIEW

The first steps in the diagnosis and treatment of a patient who is prescribed anticoagulant or antiplatelet drugs with suspected intracranial hemorrhage is standard medical stabilization along with obtaining a history specifically of the type and dose of anticoagulant drug, the duration and indication for prescription, medical comorbidities, especially those that may affect coagulation (eg, thrombocytopenia, renal failure, or liver disease), other medications that may affect anticoagulant drug metabolism, and the time of the last dose taken. One should determine if there is a history of trauma. Neurologic examination focusing on level of consciousness and detection of focal neurologic deficits is mandatory.

A noncontrast head computed tomography (CT) scan remains the gold standard for emergency assessment of pathology. A CT scan is indicated in all patients with acute spontaneous neurologic deterioration. In general, indications for CT scan in patients with TBI include any patient with Glasgow coma score of 12 or less (moderate and severe TBI) and in minor TBI (Glasgow coma score 13–15) with any of Glasgow coma score less than 15 greater than 2 hours after injury, suspected skull fracture, vomiting 2 or more times, age of at least 65 years, retrograde amnesia greater than 30 minutes, and dangerous mechanism of injury (pedestrian struck by motor vehicle, ejection from motor vehicle or fall from >3 feet or 5 stairs).[24] Basically, there are no TBI patients taking VKA, NOACs, or clopidogrel in whom a CT scan is not indicated.[25]

Bleeding may be classified as major or nonmajor, although this is less relevant in neurosurgery, since all intracranial and intraspinal bleeding that is symptomatic is major.[26]

Laboratory tests that should be obtained to assess the function of the coagulation and thrombosis pathways include those listed in **Tables 2** and **3**. Tests to assess for antiplatelet drugs include platelet number and assays of platelet function. Some commercially available assays for function include VerifyNow-ASA and VerifyNow-P2Y12 assays (Accumetrics, San Diego, California), PFA-100 (Siemens AG, Germany), and thromboelastography with platelet mapping (TEG-PM, Hemoscope Corporation, Niles, Illinois).

Dabigatran and argatroban are direct thrombin (factor II) inhibitors. Argatroban is a short-acting intravenous inhibitor mainly indicated in patients with heparin-induced thrombocytopenia. The best tests for assessing dabigatran effect are dilute thrombin time, ecarin clotting time, and ecarin chromogenic assay, but none of these are widely available. In their absence, measure the thrombin time and activated partial thromboplastin time (aPTT), since they provide a qualitative assessment of dabigatran effect. Normal thrombin time excludes any important dabigatran effect, whereas if it is elevated, this may not be therapeutically relevant. The aPTT can be normal or elevated.

Factor Xa inhibitors include rivaroxaban, apixaban, and edoxaban. Their effect can be determined by a chromogenic anti-factor Xa assay.[27]

The prothrombin time (PT) may be used for a qualitative assessment of edoxaban and rivaroxaban. A prolonged PT indicates at least a therapeutic effect of the drug. However, a therapeutic effect can also occur with a normal PT. The PT and aPTT are insensitive to apixaban therapeutic effect and can be normal under such conditions.

REVERSAL OF ANTITHROMBOTIC DRUGS

A risk/benefit assessment should be performed when considering reversal of antithrombosis drugs, because there is limited high-level evidence to support emergency reversal of antiplatelet/anticoagulant drugs; additionally, such reversal is associated with a risk of complications including thromboembolism. Even though it seems so obvious, the association of anticoagulant and antiplatelet drug use with increased morbidity and mortality after intracranial hemorrhage as reviewed previously is not well documented, and it does not follow even if there is an association, that emergent/immediate reversal of the drug effects will reduce the putative increased morbidity and mortality. Consultation with other relevant medical and surgical specialties is frequently required. The anticoagulant or antiplatelet drug should almost always be discontinued. Oral activated charcoal

Table 2
Oral antiplatelet drugs

Generic Name	Mechanism of Action	Elimination Half-Life	Reversal Strategy	Laboratory Monitoring
Acetylsalicylic acid (aspirin)	Irreversible COX inhibition	20 min, effectively 3–4 d	Platelet transfusion, desmopressin	Arachidonic acid-based testing (VerifyNow ASA), PFA
Dipyridamole	Phosphodiesterase inhibitor	10–12 h	None	None
Ticlopidine	Thienopyridine, irreversible P2Y12 receptor inhibition	4–5 d	None, consider platelet transfusion	Bleeding time, thrombin time, aPTT
Clopidogrel	Thienopyridine, irreversible P2Y12 receptor inhibition	6 h	Platelet transfusion, desmopressin	P2Y12 receptor cascade test (VerifyNow P2Y12), thrombin time, aPTT
Prasugrel	Thienopyridine, irreversible P2Y12 receptor inhibition	2–15 h	Platelet transfusion, desmopressin	P2Y12 receptor cascade test (VerifyNow P2Y12), thrombin time, aPTT
Ticagrelor	Cyclopentyltriazolopyrimidine, reversible P2Y12 receptor inhibition	7–9 h	None	None, thrombin time, aPTT

Abbreviations: aPTT, activated partial thromboplastin time; COX, cyclooxygenase; PFA, platelet function assay.

Table 3
Anticoagulant drugs

Generic Name	Mechanism of Action	Elimination Half-Life	Reversal Strategy	Laboratory Monitoring
Warfarin	Inhibition of hepatic production of vitamin K-dependent factors II, VII, IX, X, protein C, protein S	25–60 h	Vitamin K plus a PCC at weight-based dosing, sometimes dose adjusted depending on INR; if no PCC available, then recombinant factor VIIa or FFP	INR
Heparin	Activate antithrombin III leading to inhibition of factor Xa and IIa (thrombin)	30–90 min	Protamine sulfate	aPTT
Low molecular weight heparins (enoxaparin, dalteparin)	Activate antithrombin III leading to inhibition of factor Xa	Variable	Protamine sulfate, recombinant factor VIIa if protamine is contraindicated	aPTT, anti-Xa assay
Dabigatran	Direct thrombin (IIa) inhibition	12–14 h	Idarucizumab, PCC if idarucizumab not available; FFP or recombinant factor VIIa if preceding not available; hemodialysis; activated charcoal	aPTT, PFA
Rivaroxaban, edoxaban	Factor Xa inhibition	7–11 h, 10–14 h	PCC; FFP or recombinant factor VIIa if preceding not available; activated charcoal	Anti-factor Xa assay
Apixaban	Factor Xa inhibition	8–15 h	PCC; FFP or recombinant factor VIIa if preceding not available; activated charcoal	Anti-factor Xa assay

Abbreviations: FFP, fresh frozen plasma; INR, international normalized ratio; PCC, prothrombin complex concentrate.

is indicated for all oral agents if there is a history of ingestion within 2 hours of presentation, particularly for loading doses or overdoses, since it absorbs the drug and reduces gastrointestinal bioavailability.[28]

Prompt reversal of all classes of anticoagulant drugs is recommended in all patients with TBI including any patient requiring surgery and any patient with traumatic intracranial hemorrhage. Situations in which reversal can be withheld include minor TBI with normal CT scan, if the INR is less than 1.5 in patients taking VKA and in stable patients who can wait for surgery until the effect of the anticoagulant drug wears off. The latter cases would typically be those with a chronic SDH, although the balance of data again supports reversal of anticoagulation in patients with acute or chronic SDH.[29]

For patients with spontaneous ICH, reversal of anticoagulant drugs was studied in a retrospective review of 55 patients that compared various somewhat random strategies.[30] The most rapid reversal of INR was with PCC, which was associated with reduced risk of expansion of the ICH. The effect on clinical outcome was not ascertainable.

The options for reversing VKA include vitamin K, fresh frozen plasma (FFP), prothrombin complex concentrates (PCCs), and recombinant factor VIIa.[31] Vitamin K is always indicated. Administering a PCC as soon as possible is the next step. Nonactivated PCC, containing 3 (II, IX, X, negligible VII, protein C and S) or 4 factors (II, VII, IX, X, protein C and S), is the fastest, most effective method of warfarin reversal, particularly when the dose is individualized based on body weight and initial INR.[32,33] If PCCs are not available, then FFP may be used. FFP reversal will require a much higher volume infusion and is relatively deficient in factor IX and is associated with a higher chance of pulmonary edema and delayed INR reversal.[2]

Recombinant factor VIIa also has been used to reverse VKA. It was mainly studied in randomized clinical trials comparing it to placebo for reducing the incidence of hematoma growth in patients with spontaneous ICH who were not taking VKA.[34,35] In this population, factor VIIa reduced hematoma expansion but had no effect on clinical outcome, and it is not recommended to reverse VKA.[29,36]

Reversal of NOACs, while not as robustly associated with reduced ICH expansion as warfarin, should nonetheless be attempted. The first treatment for reversal of dabigatran is idarucizumab, an antibody fragment that binds unbound dabigatran. Otherwise for NOACs, available strategies are similar to those for warfarin. If idarucizumab is not available, a 4-factor PCC or activated PCC should be administered in patients taking dabigatran. Dabigatran is not protein bound and is cleared by the kidneys and hence, particularly in patients with pre-existing renal dysfunction, hemodialysis may be considered to expedite clearance.[29]

Rivaroxaban and apixaban are direct thrombin inhibitors. The PT is not useful for assessing anticoagulant effect, and hemodialysis is not helpful. The first treatment is a 4-factor PCC, with second treatment being an activated PCC.[2]

Evidence supporting reversal of antiplatelet drugs is less convincing than for anticoagulants. Although some studies have associated increased platelet inhibition with increased ICH volume expansion, and platelet transfusion within 12 hours of ictus with improved clinical outcome, others have shown no benefit with attempted reversal via platelet transfusion.[29] A randomized controlled trial of platelet transfusion in ICH patients on antiplatelet drugs found that platelet transfusion within 6 hours of presentation was associated with significantly worse clinical outcome and increased adverse events.[37] At present, the antiplatelet drug should be discontinued in general, but platelet transfusions are not recommended in patients with traumatic or spontaneous intracranial hemorrhage. If the patient requires urgent surgery before the effect of the antiplatelet drug has worn off, then some authors recommend platelet transfusion.[29] Desmopressin (DDAVP) may restore platelet function and has minimal side effects, and some guidelines recommend DDAVP for antiplatelet-related intracranial hemorrhage, which may be combined with platelet transfusion in patients undergoing surgery.[29]

Reversal of heparin is relatively easy, because it has a short half-life and is effectively bound and inactivated by intravenous protamine. The aPTT assesses the effect. Low molecular weight heparins are less effectively reversed by protamine, although this is still the main treatment. The aPTT is not useful for these drugs, and if needed, a factor Xa activity assay is better.

Recombinant tissue plasminogen activator is typically indicated in acute myocardial infarction and ischemic stroke within a short time of stroke onset. The risk of intracranial hemorrhage when administered for myocardial infarction is 0.7% and for stroke it is 3% to 9%.[31] How to reverse fibrinolysis caused by tissue plasminogen activator is based on only a few cases. Cryoprecipitate and platelet transfusions are recommended, with monitoring of fibrinogen and D-dimer concentrations.

POSTOPERATIVE RESUMPTION OF ANTITHROMBOTIC DRUGS

Resumption of anticoagulant and antiplatelet drugs after intracranial hemorrhage requires evaluating the risks of rebleeding and the potential efficacy of the drugs if they are restarted and the risks of thromboembolic complications if the drugs are not resumed. Alternatives such as inferior vena cava filters can be considered in patients with VTE. The second question is when to resume them. Grading systems should be employed to quantitate risk if they are available.[18–21] Review of such data, for example, may indicate that in some cases the risk of thromboembolic complications, such as in elderly chronic SDH patients with atrial fibrillation and a low CHA_2DS_2-VASc score, may exceed the benefits.

Patients usually suffer trauma once and have no increased risk of bleeding if an antithrombotic drug is resumed after they have recovered. The original indication for the drug should be re-evaluated but in most cases, the drug can be restarted. Chronic SDH, however, can recur spontaneously. Some literature suggests that restarting VKA 3 or more days after surgery may be safe.[38,39] The typical time to restart is 4 weeks after surgery. There are no data to inform physicians on if and when to resume NOAC. Resumption of antiplatelet agents 1 week after chronic SDH evacuation was not associated with an increase in subsequent recurrence.[40]

In patients with spontaneous ICH, there is evidence that the risk of recurrent hemorrhage is higher in patients with lobar (especially when caused by amyloid angiopathy) versus deep, with multiple cerebral microhemorrhages, older age, and apolipoprotein E e2 or e4 alleles.[36] For deep ICH, one can consider resumption of VKA, whereas in patients with nonvalvular atrial fibrillation and VKA-associated lobar ICH, resumption is not recommended. There are no data on resumption or use of NOAC in this situation. Usually the time to resume is 4 weeks after the ICH. Antiplatelet drugs can probably be resumed days after ICH, but there has to be a good indication for them.

REFERENCES

1. Writing Group Members, Mozaffarian D, Benjamin EJ, Go AS, et al. Heart disease and stroke statistics-2016 update: a report from the American Heart Association. Circulation 2016; 133(4):e38–360.

2. Tomaselli GF, Mahaffey KW, Cuker A, et al. 2017 ACC expert consensus decision pathway on management of bleeding in patients on oral anticoagulants: a report of the American College of Cardiology Task Force on Expert Consensus Decision Pathways. J Am Coll Cardiol 2017;70(24): 3042–67.

3. Furie KL, Kasner SE, Adams RJ, et al. Guidelines for the prevention of stroke in patients with stroke or transient ischemic attack: a guideline for healthcare professionals from the American Heart Association/ American Stroke Association. Stroke 2011;42(1): 227–76.

4. Lievre M, Cucherat M. Aspirin in the secondary prevention of cardiovascular disease: an update of the APTC meta-analysis. Fundam Clin Pharmacol 2010; 24(3):385–91.

5. Afshari A, Ageno W, Ahmed A, et al. European guidelines on perioperative venous thromboembolism prophylaxis: executive summary. Eur J Anaesthesiol 2018;35(2):77–83.

6. ACTIVE Writing Group of the ACTIVE Investigators, Connolly S, Pogue J, Hart R, et al. Clopidogrel plus aspirin versus oral anticoagulation for atrial fibrillation in the Atrial fibrillation Clopidogrel Trial with Irbesartan for prevention of Vascular Events (ACTIVE W): a randomised controlled trial. Lancet 2006;367(9526):1903–12.

7. Batchelor JS, Grayson A. A meta-analysis to determine the effect of preinjury antiplatelet agents on mortality in patients with blunt head trauma. Br J Neurosurg 2013;27(1):12–8.

8. Smits M, Dippel DW, Steyerberg EW, et al. Predicting intracranial traumatic findings on computed tomography in patients with minor head injury: the CHIP prediction rule. Ann Intern Med 2007;146(6): 397–405.

9. Dossett LA, Riesel JN, Griffin MR, et al. Prevalence and implications of preinjury warfarin use: an analysis of the National Trauma Databank. Arch Surg 2011;146(5):565–70.

10. Batchelor JS, Grayson A. A meta-analysis to determine the effect of anticoagulation on mortality in patients with blunt head trauma. Br J Neurosurg 2012; 26(4):525–30.

11. Baechli H, Nordmann A, Bucher HC, et al. Demographics and prevalent risk factors of chronic subdural haematoma: results of a large single-center cohort study. Neurosurg Rev 2004;27(4): 263–6.

12. Szczygielski J, Gund SM, Schwerdtfeger K, et al. Factors affecting outcome in treatment of chronic subdural hematoma in ICU patients: impact of anticoagulation. World Neurosurg 2016;92:426–33.

13. Guha D, Macdonald RL. Perioperative management of anticoagulation. Neurosurg Clin N Am 2017;28(2): 287–95.

14. Nathan S, Goodarzi Z, Jette N, et al. Anticoagulant and antiplatelet use in seniors with chronic subdural hematoma: systematic review. Neurology 2017; 88(20):1889–93.

15. Schuss P, Hadjiathanasiou A, Brandecker S, et al. Anticoagulation therapy in patients suffering from aneurysmal subarachnoid hemorrhage: influence on functional outcome-a single-center series and multivariate analysis. World Neurosurg 2017;99: 348–52.

16. Dasenbrock HH, Yan SC, Gross BA, et al. The impact of aspirin and anticoagulant usage on outcomes after aneurysmal subarachnoid hemorrhage: a nationwide inpatient sample analysis. J Neurosurg 2017;126(2):537–47.

17. Hart RG, Diener HC, Yang S, et al. Intracranial hemorrhage in atrial fibrillation patients during anticoagulation with warfarin or dabigatran: the RE-LY trial. Stroke 2012;43(6):1511–7.

18. Gage BF, Waterman AD, Shannon W, et al. Validation of clinical classification schemes for predicting stroke: results from the National Registry of Atrial Fibrillation. JAMA 2001;285(22):2864–70.

19. Lane DA, Lip GY. Use of the CHA(2)DS(2)-VASc and HAS-BLED scores to aid decision making for thromboprophylaxis in nonvalvular atrial fibrillation. Circulation 2012;126(7):860–5.

20. Pisters R, Lane DA, Nieuwlaat R, et al. A novel user-friendly score (HAS-BLED) to assess 1-year risk of major bleeding in patients with atrial fibrillation: the Euro Heart Survey. Chest 2010;138(5):1093–100.

21. Fang MC, Go AS, Chang Y, et al. A new risk scheme to predict warfarin-associated hemorrhage: the ATRIA (Anticoagulation and Risk Factors in Atrial Fibrillation) Study. J Am Coll Cardiol 2011;58(4): 395–401.

22. Bruins Slot KM, Berge E. Factor Xa inhibitors versus vitamin K antagonists for preventing cerebral or systemic embolism in patients with atrial fibrillation. Cochrane Database Syst Rev 2018;(3):CD008980.

23. Chatterjee S, Sardar P, Biondi-Zoccai G, et al. New oral anticoagulants and the risk of intracranial hemorrhage: traditional and Bayesian meta-analysis and mixed treatment comparison of randomized trials of new oral anticoagulants in atrial fibrillation. JAMA Neurol 2013;70(12):1486–90.

24. Stiell IG, Clement CM, Grimshaw JM, et al. A prospective cluster-randomized trial to implement the Canadian CT Head Rule in emergency departments. CMAJ 2010;182(14):1527–32.

25. Nishijima DK, Offerman SR, Ballard DW, et al. Risk of traumatic intracranial hemorrhage in patients with head injury and preinjury warfarin or clopidogrel use. Acad Emerg Med 2013;20(2):140–5.

26. Schulman S, Kearon C, Subcommittee on Control of Anticoagulation of the Scientific and Standardization Committee of the International Society on Thrombosis and Haemostasis. Definition of major bleeding in clinical investigations of antihemostatic medicinal products in non-surgical patients. J Thromb Haemost 2005;3(4):692–4.

27. Samuelson BT, Cuker A, Siegal DM, et al. Laboratory assessment of the anticoagulant activity of direct oral anticoagulants: a systematic review. Chest 2017;151(1):127–38.

28. James RF, Palys V, Lomboy JR, et al. The role of anticoagulants, antiplatelet agents, and their reversal strategies in the management of intracerebral hemorrhage. Neurosurg Focus 2013;34(5):E6.

29. Frontera JA, Lewin JJ 3rd, Rabinstein AA, et al. Guideline for reversal of antithrombotics in intracranial hemorrhage: a statement for healthcare professionals from the Neurocritical Care Society and Society of Critical Care Medicine. Neurocrit Care 2016;24(1):6–46.

30. Huttner HB, Schellinger PD, Hartmann M, et al. Hematoma growth and outcome in treated neurocritical care patients with intracerebral hemorrhage related to oral anticoagulant therapy: comparison of acute treatment strategies using vitamin K, fresh frozen plasma, and prothrombin complex concentrates. Stroke 2006;37(6):1465–70.

31. Vanderwerf JD, Kumar MA. Management of neurologic complications of coagulopathies. Handb Clin Neurol 2017;141:743–61.

32. Guest JF, Watson HG, Limaye S. Modeling the cost-effectiveness of prothrombin complex concentrate compared with fresh frozen plasma in emergency warfarin reversal in the United kingdom. Clin Ther 2010;32(14):2478–93.

33. van Aart L, Eijkhout HW, Kamphuis JS, et al. Individualized dosing regimen for prothrombin complex concentrate more effective than standard treatment in the reversal of oral anticoagulant therapy: an open, prospective randomized controlled trial. Thromb Res 2006;118(3):313–20.

34. Mayer SA, Brun NC, Begtrup K, et al. Recombinant activated factor VII for acute intracerebral hemorrhage. N Engl J Med 2005;352(8):777–85.

35. Mayer SA, Brun NC, Begtrup K, et al. Efficacy and safety of recombinant activated factor VII for acute intracerebral hemorrhage. N Engl J Med 2008; 358(20):2127–37.

36. Hemphill JC 3rd, Greenberg SM, Anderson CS, et al. Guidelines for the management of spontaneous intracerebral hemorrhage: a guideline for healthcare professionals from the American Heart Association/American Stroke Association. Stroke 2015;46(7):2032–60.

37. Baharoglu MI, Cordonnier C, Al-Shahi Salman R, et al. Platelet transfusion versus standard care after acute stroke due to spontaneous cerebral haemorrhage associated with antiplatelet therapy (PATCH): a randomised, open-label, phase 3 trial. Lancet 2016;387(10038):2605–13.

38. Guha D, Coyne S, Macdonald RL. Timing of the resumption of antithrombotic agents following surgical evacuation of chronic subdural hematomas: a retrospective cohort study. J Neurosurg 2016; 124(3):750–9.

39. Chari A, Clemente MT, Rigamonti D. Recommencement of anticoagulation in chronic subdural haematoma: a systematic review and meta-analysis. Br J Neurosurg 2014;28(1):2–7.

40. Torihashi K, Sadamasa N, Yoshida K, et al. Independent predictors for recurrence of chronic subdural hematoma: a review of 343 consecutive surgical cases. Neurosurgery 2008;63(6):1125–9.

Moving?

Make sure your subscription moves with you!

To notify us of your new address, find your **Clinics Account Number** (located on your mailing label above your name), and contact customer service at:

Email: journalscustomerservice-usa@elsevier.com

800-654-2452 (subscribers in the U.S. & Canada)
314-447-8871 (subscribers outside of the U.S. & Canada)

Fax number: 314-447-8029

Elsevier Health Sciences Division
Subscription Customer Service
3251 Riverport Lane
Maryland Heights, MO 63043

*To ensure uninterrupted delivery of your subscription, please notify us at least 4 weeks in advance of move.

Printed and bound by CPI Group (UK) Ltd, Croydon, CR0 4YY

08/05/2025

01864728-0001

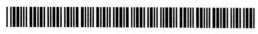